WRESTLING WITH THE ANGEL

Literary Writings and Reflections on Death, Dying and Bereavement

Kent L. Koppelman

Death, Value, and Meaning Series
Series Editor: Dale A. Lund

Baywood Publishing Company, Inc.
AMITYVILLE, NEW YORK

Copyright © 2010 by Baywood Publishing Company, Inc., Amityville, New York

All rights reserved. No part of this book may be reproduced or utilized in any form or by any means, electronic or mechanical, including photocopying, recording, or by any information storage or retrieval system, without permission in writing from the publisher. Printed in the United States of America on acid-free recycled paper.

Baywood Publishing Company, Inc.
26 Austin Avenue
P.O. Box 337
Amityville, NY 11701
(800) 638-7819
E-mail: baywood@baywood.com
Web site: baywood.com

Library of Congress Catalog Number: 2009041907
ISBN: 978-0-89503-392-5

Library of Congress Cataloging-in-Publication Data

Koppelman, Kent L.
   Wrestling with the angel : literary writings and reflections on death, dying and bereavement / Kent L. Koppelman.
      p. cm. -- (Death, value, and meaning series)
   Includes bibliographical references and index.
   ISBN 987-0-89503-392-5 (cloth : alk. paper) 1. Death--Psychological aspects. 2. Bereavement--Psychological aspects. 3. Death in literature. I. Title.
   BF789.D4K68 2010
   155.9'37--dc22

                                                2009041907

Cover art: Gauguin, Vision of the Sermon: Used with permission from *The National Gallery of Scotland*.

Dedication

To

Craig Fiedler
Teacher, Scholar, Author, Advocate, Friend

You brought the light of love and the warmth of humor to some of the coldest and darkest moments of my life.

Now you are engaged in your own fierce struggle with a foe that slipped in quietly, cloaked in cancer.

I am not able to help you as you helped me, and that has increased my misery as I watch from the sidelines.

So one thing I can do is to dedicate this book to you as an expression of my gratitude for your friendship.

As you continue your lonely and exhausting struggle, I will continue to applaud your efforts and encourage you; I will continue to shout out words of love and of hope.

And as long as you can still hear me, I will keep shouting.

(Craig Fiedler died on Sunday, January 4, 2009.)

Table of Contents

BAYWOOD'S FREE GIFT TO READERS OF
WRESTLING WITH THE ANGEL vi

FOREWORD vii
ACKNOWLEDGMENTS xiii

PART 1: Death and Loss

CHAPTER 1: Loss: An Unexpected Death 3

CHAPTER 2: Mortality: A Matter of Life and Death 19

PART 2: Responding to an Unexpected Death

CHAPTER 3: Bereavement: Becoming a Survivor 51

CHAPTER 4: Reconciliation: Living with an Absence 63

PART 3: Responding to Expected Deaths

CHAPTER 5: Bereavement: Expecting Death 81

CHAPTER 6: Awareness: Promoting the Quality of Life 101

PART 4: Approaching the End of Life

CHAPTER 7: Growing Old: Walking through the Valley 117

CHAPTER 8: Anticipation: Preparing for Death 127

AFTERWORD: Final Thoughts 145
INDEX 147

BAYWOOD'S FREE GIFT TO READERS OF *WRESTLING WITH THE ANGEL*

Lucky Man: A Matter of Life and Death

Written by Kent L. Koppelman with Paul Dominic Heckman
Produced by Jan Koppelman

*A one-act play originally performed for the
International Death, Grief and Bereavement Conference
at La Crosse, Wisconsin, June 2007*

THE PLAYERS

Death	**Kent L. Koppelman**
Adam Mensch	**Paul Dominic Heckman**
Narrator	**Tess Koppelman**
Original Musical Composition	**Jan Koppelman**

SYNOPSIS: A middle-aged man named Adam Mensch receives a surprise visit from the Angel of Death. Mensch protests that he is not ready to go, but the Angel insists that his time has come. The play presents their discussion before Adam agrees to leave with his visitor. To provide some insight into the nature of the collaboration between the two authors who created this one-act play, you are invited to read each author's perspective on the play.

Koppelman's Perspective: This play consists of a desperate dialogue between a man who has lived what Socrates called an "unexamined life" and an Angel of Death who has a certain amount of compassion but who has a job to do. While Adam tries to convince the Angel that he should be given more time before leaving this life, the Angel tries to explain to Adam that his arguments are pointless because death comes when it will come. Their discussion addresses questions of philosophy, theology, and religious beliefs while addressing the purpose of life, the meaning of death, the existence of a soul and, of course, God. The Angel ultimately answers one question that allows Adam to accept his fate.

Heckman's Perspective: According to several reliable reports, another man has, in the vernacular "made the grade." Doctors Allen, Blake, Crane, Dickenson, France, Keats, Schweitzer, and Swift have all weighed in with their own unique take on the incident. One Mr. Adam Mensch had, in fact, been joined in discussions bordering on bargaining, begging, and negotiation, before ultimately accepting the opposition perspective. Mensch at times parried masterfully; at others he resorted to the age-old, "Wait." Or the tired chestnut, "But I have questions." Such attempts, as usual, designed or created, were met with amusement and satire. Mensch's position did nothing to override biology or history.

Format: MP3
Duration: 29 minutes

Foreword

Within a few months after my 19-year-old son died in a traffic accident, I began to revise my grief journal into a manuscript that became *The Fall of a Sparrow: Of Death and Dreams and Healing* (1994). I wrote it in part out of frustration from reading several books and finding few, especially those written by grieving fathers, that helped me to deal with this loss in any meaningful way. Writing *Sparrow* was in part personal therapy, and in part an attempt to offer assistance to others who were struggling with the unexpected loss of a loved one, especially a child.

Writing the book was helpful for me, but it did not resolve the issues in my ongoing effort to be at peace with the absence of my son on a daily basis. Although it was more sporadic, I continued to write essays and some poetry about my thoughts and experiences with death—a close friend died, then my sister, and my parents. Over the years, four of my essays were published. In the fall of 2006 I wrote a one-act play about the Angel of Death coming for a man who was not ready to leave and insists that he should not be taken yet. A friend and skilled writer, Paul Dominic Heckman, assisted me in revising the play, and we performed it at an annual Death and Bereavement Conference. The audience responded enthusiastically, and after the performance several people requested copies of the script. This was the genesis of the book you now have before you. I began to organize and revise my published and unpublished writing, and I worked on some new material, especially an essay with the tentative title, "Wrestling with the Angel."

In addition to my own writing, I have collected numerous excerpts from poetry and prose over the years, which included a significant number on issues related to death, grief, and bereavement. They represent part of what I think of as "wisdom literature" on these topics. My interest in collecting excerpts from literature stems from growing up in rural Nebraska in the 1950s and attending a one-room school. For all its drawbacks, there were advantages for a child who loved to read. Our elementary readers included authors such as Robert Burns, Edgar Allan Poe, and William Wordsworth, who would be considered too literary (meaning too difficult for children to read) by today's standards. Students read aloud, so when I was younger I would listen to the language of the literature being read by the older students and was captivated by these literary descriptions of human fears, joys, despairs, and triumphs. In high school and in college I continued to read compelling literature, including some that addressed human experiences and beliefs about death, grief, and immortality.

Approaching the age of 30, I enrolled in a PhD program in education and began to read a wide range of nonfiction, while continuing to read literature. In addition to gaining knowledge, I also appreciated those authors who could make a comment that compelled attention. Others might have said the same thing, but this author said it in a way that made it memorable. Whenever I came across such quotations, I began to write them down and save them. With the advent of computers, I transferred these pages to a file that now contains over 300 pages of quotations. It was from this collection on a multitude of topics that I selected excerpts and quotations for this book, which I consider to be good examples of wisdom literature on issues of death and dying, grief and bereavement.

Some of the quotations are well-known passages that are often cited, while others are relatively obscure. Some can be found in prose from which another passage is more frequently quoted. For example, most people are familiar with the phrase "for whom the bell tolls," if not from its actual source then as the title of an Ernest Hemingway novel (that became a movie). People who recognize the phrase may know that it comes from the poet John Donne (1951); however, it is not from a poem but from his *Meditation 17*:

> No man is an island entire of itself; every man is a piece of the continent, a part of the main. If a clod be washed away by the sea, Europe is the less, as well as if a promontory were, as well as if a manor of thy friend's or thine own were. Any man's death diminishes me, because I am involved in mankind, and therefore never send to know for whom the bell tolls; it tolls for thee. (pp. 340-341)

Earlier in that same meditation, Donne writes another passage that is as compelling and inspirational, if not more so, than the more famous passage:

> All mankind is of one author, and is one volume; when one man dies, one chapter is not torn out of the book, but translated into a better language; and every chapter must be so translated. God employs several translators; some pieces are translated by age, some by sickness, some by war, some by justice; but God's hand is in every translation, and his hand shall bind up all our scattered leaves again for that library where every book shall lie open to one another. (p. 340)

I would like to see someone create a book filled with such wisdom literature, not merely a book of quotations (we already have those) but passages that reveal profound insights from diverse authors on human experiences and perceptions of death, grief, and bereavement. Passages like the ones above have been the catalyst for my own thinking and writing about grief and bereavement. A few scattered showers of prose became a downpour after my son died, and after I had written a rough draft of *Sparrow*, I selected quotations from my collection to begin each chapter.

As noted earlier, four of the essays in this book were previously published, and I want to express my appreciation to the publishers for allowing the inclusion of these essays in this book. "Emerging from the Anguish: A Father's Experience with Loss and Grief" Koppelman (2000) cited in an anthology of writing on men's grief experiences entitled *Men Coping with Grief*. Two essays were published in the journal *Illness, Crisis & Loss*: "The Dance of Grief" Koppelman (1999) describing rituals and actions to promote healing; "The Culture of Life" Koppelman (2005) suggested that an awareness of death may be necessary for people to develop a genuine reverence for life. "For Those Who Stand and Wait" Koppelman (2003) an essay selected for the anthology *Making Sense of Death*, describes my attempts to be reconciled to my son's death.

In reviewing the writing to be included in this book, eight themes emerged that were related to death, grief, and bereavement, and that seemed appropriate as a framework for this book. For each of the eight chapters there is an introductory essay exploring the theme, and throughout each introductory essay the reader will encounter several boxed texts with excerpts from the wisdom literature on death, grief, and bereavement. After each introductory essay there is a poem and then another piece of writing that addresses the theme for that chapter. This writing is usually an essay, but also includes a one-act play, a short story and, in the chapter about the loss of my sister, father, and mother, there are four poems. When the manuscript was almost finished, I decided to add a final page of quotations at the end consisting of comments attributed to people as they were about to die, and in some cases the comment allegedly represents their final words.

This description explains how the book was created, and the variety of writing is intended to illustrate how our feelings about such issues as aging and mortality, loss and grief can be expressed in different ways using different approaches to say what needs to be said. In Part 1, the first chapter describes the beginning of my personal journey with grief. People in my life had died—grandmothers and uncles and aunts. In every case they were older people whose long and full lives provided a sense of closure to lighten the burden of the loss. My real grief journey began with the death of my son. This encounter with his unexpected death brought unanswered and unanswerable questions and at times a sense of anger reflected in early poems. The chapter concludes with the first essay that I wrote after Jason's death. The second chapter explores the theme of mortality, because becoming genuinely conscious of death makes one conscious of one's own mortality, and that represents a critical point in a person's life. Leo Tolstoy insisted that human beings have not really begun to think until they had accepted their mortality. A consciousness of mortality often leads to a religious faith and may include certain beliefs about good and evil, God and the devil, so this seemed to be the best place to include my favorite shape poem—a monologue from the devil presented in the form of a question mark, the shape emphasizing the role of doubt in the search for faith. The one-act play concerns a man who was not conscious of death and had given no thought to his mortality until he was forced to confront the issue when the Angel of Death came for him.

In Part 2, the chapters examine two aspects of the grief journey. The first chapter describes a survivor searching for ways to heal from an unexpected death, and the next chapter discusses the attempt to reach a form of reconciliation with that death. Part 3 begins by examining responses to an expected death due to terminal illness or to deteriorating health. Most people will have friends or family members who succumb to an illness such as cancer or provide care for elderly parents or grandparents who struggle with health problems. When we know that someone will die soon, that expectation does not eliminate our feelings for the person or our sense of loss when the person dies, but it does change the context for that death and the way people respond to it. The chapter concludes with poetry written in the aftermath of such expected deaths. After a loved one dies, death may become an ongoing presence in one's life, but chapter 6 argues that an awareness of death does not have to lead to despair but can become a critical factor for enhancing the quality of one's life.

In Part 4, the content of the first chapter reflects the bittersweet quality often found in writing about aging. As we age we find ourselves losing and gaining—losing some physical and mental abilities but gaining a better perspective on life because of our experiences. Wisdom says to savor the days behind us and look forward to the days before us while still paying attention to the present—the today that will soon be another yesterday. Having just turned 60, I am better able to appreciate this feeling, and it is reflected in the song lyrics included here. As an American, I live in a culture emulating youth and passionate sexuality, so the short story is a gentle refutation of the bias of the culture. It suggests that what is ultimately important are the relationships we maintain over time, and that love is a gift beyond value since it provides us with the genuine passion necessary to sustain a human being.

Finally, the last chapter discusses why we need to be prepared for death and what such preparation involves; the essay for this chapter was written especially for this book. *Wrestling with the Angel* represents the culmination of several years of thinking about death, loss, grief, and bereavement. In describing my struggle "with the angel," this essay brings the book full circle, because the angel in its title alludes to the character of the Angel of Death from the one-act play in Part 1, who appears before a very mortal and very unprepared Adam Mensch to take him away.

The final page of the book consists of comments from various people as they approached death, and all of comments demonstrate that no one can give us the answers to our questions. In that sense these quotations illustrate a fundamental assumption of this book. With regard to all of the issues addressed, readers must be content to ask questions and select those answers that make the most sense to them, and those answers will differ for each individual. My own response is to be hopeful—for humanity in general—that we can find satisfying answers.

I became a teacher because I wanted to make a difference in people's lives—to offer not only knowledge but hope and compassion to counter the difficulties in life. I don't know that I have succeeded, but my actions have attempted to reflect the Greek proverb: "A society grows great when old men plant trees whose shade they know they shall never sit in." My feelings still have the power they had in my youth, but my body tells me that I am aging. My students began perceiving me as old years ago, whereas to those older than me I have not gained that distinction yet. So as I move into the status of being considered an old man by larger numbers of people, this book represents another tree among several that I have planted. And like the others, I hope there will be some, perhaps only a few, perhaps more, who will find comfort within the quiet shade provided by its leaves.

REFERENCES

Donne, J. (1951). Meditation 17. In A. Witherspoon (Ed.), *The college survey of English literature.* New York: Harcourt, Brace & World.

Koppelman, K. (1994). *The fall of a sparrow: Of death, dreams, and healing.* Amityville, NY: Baywood.

Koppelman, K. (1999). The dance of grief. In G. Cox & T. Gongaware (Eds.), *Illness, Crisis & Loss, 7*(3), 213-217. Sage Publications.

Koppelman, K. (2000). Emerging from the anguish: A father's experience with loss and grief. In D. Lund (Ed.), *Men coping with grief* (pp. 85-95). Amityville, NY: Baywood.

Koppelman, K. (2003). For those who stand and wait. In G. Cox & R. Bendiksen (Eds.), *Making sense of death* (pp. 45-52), Amityville, NY: Baywood.

Koppelman, K. (2005). The culture of life. In G. Cox & T. Gongaware (Eds.), *Illness, Crisis & Loss, 13*(4) 351-357. Sage Publications.

Acknowledgments

There are many people whose encouragement, support, and suggestions contributed to this book. I am grateful to Paul Heckman for reading a draft of my one-act play "Lucky Man" and offering many additions and revisions to make it better. When we performed the play together at a bereavement conference, the enthusiastic reception from the audience was the catalyst for writing this book. I also want to express my appreciation to Gerry Cox, Greg Wegner, Craig Fiedler and my sister, Sally Sinclair; all read a draft of the manuscript and made many suggestions and positive comments. Including poetry and fiction was a departure from my past writing, so I needed to be reassured that this writing was as meaningful as my essays. My good friend Craig Fiedler was especially helpful in making a number of suggestions even as he struggled with his fatal illness. There are no words to express how much I miss him.

I am deeply grateful to my sister Sally for allowing me to include her poem "Swing Time," and to my wife, Jan, for sharing her thoughts about the manuscript and for suggesting the Paul Gauguin painting for the cover of this book. Thanks also to Dale Lund for his encouragement, and to Julie Krempa at Baywood for her tireless efforts. Last but certainly not least, Bobbi Olszewski deserves recognition for her work and her patience with me as we brought this book forward to see the light of day. Everyone named here made this a better book, but I remain responsible for its flaws.

PART 1

Death and Loss

Dirge Without Music

*I am not resigned to the shutting away of loving hearts in the
  hard ground.*
So it is, and so it will be, for so it has been, time out of mind:
Into the darkness they go, the wise and the lovely. Crowned
With lilies and with laurel they go; but I am not resigned.

Lovers and thinkers, into the earth with you.
Be one with the dull, the indiscriminate dust.
A fragment of what you felt, of what you knew,
A formula, a phrase remains, – but the best is lost.

*The answers quick and keen, the honest look, the laughter,
  the love, –*
They are gone. They are gone to feed the roses. Elegant and curled
*Is the blossom. Fragrant is the blossom. I know. But I do not
  approve.*
*More precious was the light in your eyes than all the roses in
  the world.*

Down, down, down into the darkness of the grave
Gently they go, the beautiful, the tender, the kind;
Quietly they go, the intelligent, the witty, the brave.
I know. But I do not approve. And I am not resigned.

Edna St. Vincent Millay

Copyright © 1928, 1955 by Edna St. Vincent Millay
and Norma Millay Ellis. Reprinted by permission of
Elizabeth Barnett, Literary Executor
The Millay Society.

CHAPTER 1

Loss:
An Unexpected Death

Every one can master a grief but he that has it.
William Shakespeare

At some point we all contemplate our own mortality, but I never expected to be confronted with the mortality of my own child. When my 19-year-old son died in a car accident, my sunny world was shrouded in darkness. Despite the chaos of emotions, I managed to get through the next few days as if in a trance, doggedly plodding along beside my wife as we took care of funeral arrangements and then endured the funeral itself. It was good to have family and friends there, embracing us and offering their love and sympathy, but the reason for their presence was lying in a coffin at the front of the room, and that took precedence over everything else.

During the reception following the funeral, I had to be the host, but this was not a festive event, not a celebration but a farewell party. And the farewell was forever. I was grateful for the compassion of the people who were there, but I was not ready to say "farewell" to my son in any meaningful way. I would spend the next 2 decades finding ways to say farewell to him, going to his grave at least once a week, just standing there—sometimes talking, sometimes silent.

Part of the grieving process was to write in a journal, expressing random thoughts and feelings. In addition, I read books written about grief, both personal and professional accounts, to learn from the experiences of others or from their collective experience as reported in research. There seemed so little written from a father's perspective that I considered writing such a book, and eventually I did. Its publication did not resolve these feelings of grief, but it helped to move me further along in the process. It felt good to believe that something came from Jason's death, something that might be helpful to others, something to inject even a modicum of sense into this senseless tragedy.

It is hard to accept the loss of a loved one after they have been a presence in your life for so many years, especially if they were young and you had expected them to be in your life for many more years to come. I have heard that people who have lost an arm or a leg say they can still feel the missing limb as though it were still attached. I have the same feeling about the loss of my child. For several months after his death, something that would have interested Jason would happen, and I would think about telling Jason, until I remembered that he was gone. The British poet William Wordsworth (1936) captured this experience perfectly:

> Surprised by joy—impatient as the Wind
> I turned to share the transport—Oh! with whom
> But Thee, deep buried in the silent tomb. (p. 204)

As time passed I remembered sooner and stopped making this mistake. Perhaps it was all those visits to the cemetery that reinforced the image of his grave, and therefore his death, so firmly in my consciousness. Yet I continued to think of Jason, sometimes by choice, sometimes surprised by moments during certain activities that would remind me of him. Jason's ambition was to make movies. After his death I often went to movies, and at the end of certain films might speculate: "Jason would have liked this movie," or "If he had lived, this is the sort of movie Jason would have made." Such thoughts prolonged my relationship with my son, providing him a space in my life. It was the only kind of immortality I could give him—that of a father's love and remembrance.

> But, O the heavy change, now thou art gone,
> Now thou art gone, and never must return!
> *John Milton*

After my book was published, I continued to write about grieving. These emotions cannot be bound up in a volume and dispensed with, even if I had wished for it. And I didn't wish for it. By the end of the book I had realized that the persistence of ongoing pain over Jason's death was a reflection of my love for him, and it was one way to keep him with me. I had also recognized that the grief experience initiated by an unexpected death was a lengthy process of saying goodbye.

Saying goodbye did not mean no longer loving Jason, even though expressing that love now exacted a painful price. Yet I suspect most parents are willing to pay that price.

> Rest in soft peace, and ask'd say here doth lye
> Ben Jonson's best piece of poetrie.
> (*Ben Jonson's epitaph on his son's gravestone*)

For parents, loving a child is always connected to other emotions, including negative ones such as fear, anxiety, and frustration. When Jason first encountered other children teasing him at school, it hurt his feelings. This was especially true in middle school when he was subjected to verbal and physical abuse. Whenever we talked about it, I felt his frustration and the suffering, and I also felt the rage of an impotent father, unable to end the abuse. I did what I could to assuage his feelings and make his way smoother. It is all any parent can do.

With his death, most of the anxiety and frustration ended, replaced by the dull, numbing pain of his absence, which was inextricably intertwined with a father's ongoing love. On those occasions at the cemetery when I stand next to his grave talking, it is not because of a belief that he can hear me but because it is the only part of a conversation with him that I have the power to create. I have never felt his presence there. Yet I still describe what I've been doing or discuss things that have happened at home or at work—ordinary, everyday items of conversation. When it is time to leave I always say goodbye, and often add, "I love you, Jason." The longing embodied in this parting comment is reflected in these lines expressing Tennyson's (1959) longing:

> But O for the touch of a vanish'd hand,
> And the sound of a voice that is still. (p. 397)

Not being able to feel that touch or hear that voice does not prevent the desire for those things. The poem called "The Lost Day" describes the bitterness of such frustrated desires. I cannot remember the reason why I wrote it. Perhaps on a day after reading newspaper accounts of young men Jason's age committing robbery, rape, or murder, and wondering why they were alive while my son was dead. It is a poem about betrayal and bitter disappointment. Grief has not been "mastered." There is no resolution, and there can be no resolution when raw wounds from a loss still throb with pain. The poem simply reports something painful that happened, something that could not be prevented, and the only recourse is to find a way to live with the pain and the suffering.

"Emerging from the Anguish" was the first essay I wrote following the publication of *Sparrow*. The essay borrows heavily from the book, but it also includes experiences that occurred after the book was published. It presents a concise statement about the feelings of grief in the wake of my son's death. It describes not only events surrounding this unexpected death but some conscious efforts to search for ways to grieve this loss and to live with the consequences of this death.

The excerpts from wisdom literature included in boxed texts throughout this essay are all about unexpected deaths. John Milton uses simple language to speak of his unexpected loss and of the permanent absence from his life. Being young, loved, or beautiful—death is oblivious to human assumptions and desires about who should have a long life. Ben Jonson mourns the loss of what he expected his son to become, while Shakespeare has a character mourning the son that was. Shakespeare's son Hamnet died as he was writing "The Life and Death of King John," and in the powerful words he writes for Constance, the grieving mother of the dead boy, there is no better expression of a parent's grief.

> Grief fills the room up of my absent child,
> Lies in his bed, walks up and down with me,
> Puts on his pretty looks, repeats his words,
> Remembers me of all his gracious parts,
> Stuffs out his vacant garments with his form:
> Then have I reason to be fond of grief.
> 									William Shakespeare

The Lost Day

Today was a day that should have died in bed,

So still, no one would know that it was dead.

"So soon the day has passed," we might have said.

But then it came, inflicting pain instead,

    And so I hate today.

Today came costumed, hiding harm; I read

The malice in its mocking mask. I bled

Inside from silent wounds, and though I shed

No tears, I drank the wine (without the bread),

    And so, I hate today.

I did not greet the day; its boldness bred

An awful memory—pale lips, once red,

When kissed they chilled my lips like kissing lead,

Warm hands caressed your unresponsive head.

    So still, I hate today.

EMERGING FROM THE ANGUISH:
A FATHER'S EXPERIENCE WITH LOSS AND GRIEF

> I see a schoolboy when I think of him,
> With face and nose pressed to a sweet-shop window,
> For certainly he sank into his grave
> His senses and his heart unsatisfied.
>
> W. B. Yeats

When the call came on the evening of September 13, 1989, it was after 11:00. My wife answered the phone. It was the Houston County Sheriff. Jason, our 19-year-old son, had been in a car accident and was being taken to Lutheran Hospital. The sheriff was calling from his car phone and the tone of his voice suggested that this was serious. The ambulance was turning into the hospital parking lot as we arrived. Jan got out of the car quickly, and I watched my wife run to the ambulance backing up to the emergency room doors. I did not run. I walked as fast as I could, trying to keep calm, trying not to let my worst fears take over. Perhaps it was Jan's brief glimpse of Jason that made her think he was dead. While I sat in a private waiting room, hoping, Jan was in the bathroom trying to overcome her nausea. I desperately repeated words like "sustained (an injury)" or even "seriously injured" or even "maimed." No matter how ugly those words seemed, at that moment they sounded better than "dead."

When the doctor finally came into the room, she spoke simply, directly. She said Jason was in an accident, and he "didn't make it." Jan took the news more calmly than I because she had prepared herself for such a statement. I had not, and I was overwhelmed with agony. Large tears splashed down my cheeks as I groaned and bent over and groaned again. I could barely hear Jan and the doctor talking. It took several minutes before I could regain some control.

The doctor asked if we wanted to see Jason's body. We did. A few minutes later we were escorted to the room where Jason's body lay. They had cleaned him up as best they could, some dried blood remained around the fingernails and someone had placed a blue shower cap on his head, presumably to hide the badly damaged skull. The doctor had explained that Jason died instantly from a severe head injury that occurred when the car flipped over onto its top.

Jan went to his right side and I to his left. My stubborn optimism refused to accept the pronouncement of his death; walking down the hall I kept thinking of the miracle of Lazarus. At Jason's side I clutched his hand and squeezed as hard as I could as if I could infuse some of my warmth, some of my life into him. Feeling how cold his palm was and staring at his familiar face with the unfamiliar sight of no breath blowing softly between parted lips, I was forced to acknowledge that my son was dead.

The pain was so intense I don't know how I could have tolerated it had it not been for the numbness. My entire body felt numb. In my brain the numbness was like a soft buzz of radio static (the volume turned low). Jan and I touched Jason's body, despite how cold and lifeless it felt. We touched and kissed him and told him we loved him. It made no sense, but neither did his death. We had to express our love even though his ears could not hear nor could his body feel our caresses. This was the beginning of a long grieving process that I only understood later as one of saying goodbye to my son.

No one is prepared for the death of their child, but I was especially overwhelmed by the myriad of decisions that had to be made. Jan and I met with the funeral director to discuss the funeral. What Bible verses . . . what music selections . . . who would give the eulogy? What clothes would Jason want to be buried in? Would he care? I didn't know all the answers, but I did know that Jason didn't want to die, not ever, and certainly not at 19. We had to select a coffin, wandering aimlessly amid the wood and metal cylinders. We had to pick out lots at the cemetery. Should we buy three lots or two? Would Tess understand why we would only want to buy three? We couldn't take the chance so we bought four. We were told we could resell the lot if we didn't need it. We hoped we would not need it, but hope was a hollow word on this day. We were about to bury our son.

For several days the buzzing in my brain continued and the numbness bore down on my body like a load of cement. In some ways this was good. The numbness helped me to get through the public visitation and the funeral, but it was draining me of energy. I seemed to be moving slowly, reinforced by the sensation of walking many fathoms below the surface the ocean. Every step, every thought required enormous effort. Although I was not sleeping well, that was not the reason for this feeling. I had gone without sleep before, and I knew how that felt. This was different. Every day at midafternoon I was exhausted, hardly able to function.

A week later I was still struggling with this burden, but returned to work. As a college professor, my work schedule was "staggered" throughout the day, and I managed to stagger through it. There were committee meetings, papers to grade, and lesson plans to write for classes on Monday evenings and late afternoon on Tuesdays, Wednesdays, and Thursdays. This schedule gave me time to go home and rest before each class, and after class I always felt drained. Teaching has always required considerable energy because in my classes students discuss sensitive social issues such as sexism, racism, and homophobia. Students have always appreciated the enthusiasm I bring to the classroom, but now I was using energy to blot out a piece of reality during classroom time. This was also true when I was in my office advising students, attending committee meetings, or observing a student teacher and meeting with the supervisor.

Sometimes people offered consolation by talking to me about the accident or telling me of other families that had experienced similar tragedies. Although they meant well, such conversations made it more difficult for me at work. On campus I needed to focus on the task to be done. I did not need to be reminded of my pain or anyone else's pain. The people who helped me the most were those who simply said how sorry they were, and some would give me a hug. That helped. When you are struggling with despair, you need people to say they care about you, and you need to know that they mean it. Even after a full week back at work, my body felt as if the force of gravity had been doubled.

It was a Wednesday morning when I awoke again at 5:00, just as I had done every morning for the past week. Lack of sleep was part of the reason I lacked energy, so if I could sleep a little longer each morning I thought I could function more effectively. In desperation I folded my hands and prayed. It was a prayer whispered in the dark by a man of little faith who freely confessed his doubts. I prayed to have the burden lifted, not just to alleviate my burden, but because I had a family that needed me. Afterwards, I thought I would lie in bed for a few more minutes and then get up. Unlike the previous mornings, I fell back asleep and had a dream.

In the dream I saw Jason and his two closest friends. Their conversation was mundane, trivial, normal—so normal I was briefly convinced that this was reality and Jason's death was simply a horrible nightmare. During the dream I felt a powerful wave of emotion—joy, relief, perhaps even a kind of ecstasy—as it raced through my body. It wasn't long before I realized that there were too many things happening that were not consistent with reality. I reluctantly accepted the conclusion that I was dreaming, but I wanted to take advantage of this illusion to satisfy my desire to hug Jason and tell him how much I loved him. When I moved toward him, I woke up. It was disappointing to be denied such a simple pleasure in my own dream. After I awoke I described the dream to Jan, and as I talked, I wept.

The effect of this dream was dramatic. I graded papers all morning and realized by the end of the morning that I was not feeling so tired. I went for my usual noon swim and came home still feeling energetic. Since the accident I had usually been too tired to continue working by this point in the day, so I would lay on the couch resting before going to teach. Instead I continued working until it was time to leave for class. I had no trouble mustering the energy and enthusiasm required for teaching, and time passed quickly. After class I came home for supper and was surprised that I was not feeling absolutely exhausted. Even before the accident I would usually come home from class feeling tired, but I felt fine. I even worked at the computer for 2 hours before relaxing for a couple of hours and then going to bed. The next day I woke up at a more normal time, and all day I functioned as I had before the accident. From that point on I had good days and bad days, but I would never again experience the level of energy I had on the day of the dream.

A few weeks later I went to the clinic for my annual physical examination, and in the conversation with my doctor I asked if he could explain how I could experience such fatigue before the dream and have so much energy on the day after the dream. He said the medical profession still had much to learn about the brain and brain functioning, but my fatigue sounded like the symptoms of clinical depression that studies say is chemically induced in the brain. He said it was possible for a dream to stimulate a chemical reaction in the brain that could counteract the chemicals causing the depression. I don't know if this is what happened to me; I only know that after the dream I was able to return to a semblance of normality in my daily life.

For some time afterwards, if I was in a conversation with a parent who had lost a child, I would ask if they had dreamed about that child. Every one of the men I talked with had a dream where they saw their child again, sometimes weeks later, even months later, but they all agreed that it was an important part of their grieving process. By contrast, I have also talked to women who lost a child and none of them had such a dream. I don't know if this is a consistent difference between men and women. If this is a difference, perhaps it is because women usually spend more time with their children so they have enough memories to satisfy the need to remember and cherish the child. Perhaps for men such dreams are an anguished effort to expand an inadequate memory base. Whatever the reason, I am grateful that my dream gave me an opportunity to see Jason again. It was the first step of a long journey toward becoming reconciled with this sudden, unexpected death that had transformed the landscape of my world.

My wife's first opportunity to say goodbye occurred at the funeral. Jan and I had shared our feelings of grief with each other from the beginning. In a conversation a few days after friends and family had returned home, Jan explained her emotional dilemma at the funeral.

She kept thinking about Jason lying in the coffin; even though he was not alive, this was all she had left of him. She didn't know how she would be able to leave the cemetery, to leave Jason behind.

During the funeral, Jan and I sat next to Tess, our 13-year-old daughter, in the front row of a section reserved for family. Other family members sat behind us. To our right was a door with a hearse parked on the other side to take Jason's coffin to the cemetery. The funeral began with recorded organ music that was dreadful; Jason would have hated it. At that moment a scraping sound seemed to come from the door leading to the parking lot. Perhaps the wind was gusting outside; I considered walking over to the door to be certain that it was closed. Suddenly the door blew open, banging against the outside wall as if a child had just burst through, anxious to get outside and enjoy the warm September day. For Jan, the door incident assured her that Jason was not in the coffin, that he had listened to that music as long as he could, but he then had to get away from it, so he had left, abruptly, neglecting to close the door. Believing that this was what had just happened made it possible for her to go to the cemetery and to leave after the ceremony, to leave the body to be buried.

When the door blew open, I had the same reaction as Jan, that it was Jason's spirit leaving, but my rational mind intruded, telling me not to indulge in such supernatural thinking. So I considered more practical explanations, such as a strong gust of wind, but when the mourners stood by the grave at the cemetery, I watched mosquitoes float lazily up and land on the front of my shirt. There was not even a gentle breeze to disturb their flight. There is still no obvious explanation for what happened, but I continue to believe that Jason's spirit forced that door open. He never liked funerals anyway, so how much more would he have disliked being at his own funeral. A sudden death gives survivors few meaningful choices, but this is a choice that has helped me to heal.

Although I had not read death and dying literature thoroughly, I had read enough to know some potential consequences during the aftermath of a traumatic death. What was surprising was how many common actions or reactions I did *not* experience. One reaction I had read about was anger, and I was prepared to feel anger at Jason for dying, for being careless while he was driving. That did not happen. I worried that my marriage might suffer, that my family might even fall apart under the burden of this tragedy. That did not happen. I was concerned about being so distracted by grief that I would not function as effectively at work. That did not happen. In each case, I think I know why.

The summer before Jason's accident, I had an opportunity to teach at a summer institute in Europe. Jason insisted he wanted to get a summer job and stay home, so Jan and Tess joined me to spend several weeks in Europe. Jason was living at home and he agreed to take care of the lawn. When we came home in mid-August, Jason had just mowed the lawn and it looked fine. Going through the stacks of mail that came during our absence, a letter from the "Weed Commissioner" said he had received complaints of weeds "four to five feet high;" if the lawn wasn't mowed soon, the city would do it and send me the bill. When I confronted Jason with the letter he simply shrugged and said, "I don't do weeds." At that moment I was too busy to discuss this with him, but as the day went on I was unable to work up a sense of "righteous wrath." That surprised me, and I could only conclude that deep inside some part of me had apparently decided to accept Jason as he was, warts and all.

In discussing this incident with a friend, he congratulated me, saying it was a sign of my maturation as a parent. I'm not so sure, but I believe this acceptance was the reason for my inability to be angry with Jason, and there were reasons to be angry. The accident occurred on a cloudless night, no bad weather or road problems. Jason was apparently not paying attention as he approached a curve in the road and drove the car onto the shoulder. He lost control of the car and it went into the ditch, flipping onto its top and his skull was crushed. The accident was clearly his fault, but I could not be angry with him. Jason had many good qualities and deserved to be loved for them. He also had flaws, one of which was a tendency to be careless, not to focus on the task at hand, especially if the task was uninteresting or mundane. For one brief moment, this became a fatal flaw.

All of us have flaws and make mistakes. As one woman said, "If everyone died each time he did something stupid there would be no one left on the planet." Because I had accepted Jason, flaws included, I could not be angry with him about the weeds, not even about the accident. It was just a case of Jason being Jason, probably driving a bit too fast, certainly being a bit careless and not paying attention. He should not have had to pay such a high price for such a minor flaw in his character, but he did.

The times I have felt anger have usually been when encountering people who mouth pious nonsense about God calling Jason home. Some people seem to have a perception of a kindly, anthropomorphic god with a flowing white beard who sits on a throne in heaven and says, "I really like (that person). Bring (him or her) to me." Among many absurdities of such a vision is that in this case God would have had to say, "Bring Jason to me and don't botch the job. Kill him good and proper. I don't want him lingering on a respirator. I suggest you flip his car over and smash his brains all over the place. That should do it." I am appalled that people could actually believe in such a ridiculous and ultimately brutal concept of God.

For a time I felt some anger toward God, but it never became intense, because I have never been certain that God exists. But at times I thought, "If there is a God, He has to bear some responsibility for the death of my son." After all, God is omnipotent. What is the good of having power if you can't use it to stop something tragic or senseless from happening? While searching through several different translations of the Bible for the passage about the sparrow to include in my manuscript, I initially selected a translation that said "not one sparrow falls to the ground without your father's *consent*" because I wanted to blame God for what had happened. As time passed, I picked up the King James version once again and decided to use this version: "one of them shall not fall on the ground *without* your father." The only God I can imagine is a God who suffers with us, who shares our pain. A God who inflicts suffering is not worthy of belief.

My relationship with Jan and Tess has been affected by Jason's death, but it has not torn our family apart. Perhaps the way Jason died was the critical factor. It might have been different if Jan or Tess or I had been in the car with Jason and survived. It's easy to believe that we would have been grateful that anyone survived, but I can also imagine the bitter feelings and accusations any of us might have harbored. Would we have overcome such feelings? I cannot be certain of that. I can also imagine the guilt I would have felt if I had been in the car and survived the accident, even if Jason had been driving. No matter how rational one tries to be, rationality does not always take precedence over powerful and often irrational feelings of guilt that often arise under such tragic circumstances. Jason spared us from that. He died alone.

Instead of blaming each other, we focused on helping each other. It was strange how consistently Jan was able to be strong when I felt weak and how I was able to be strong when she felt weak. From the beginning we seemed to take over for each other as if working in "shifts," a reflection of the strength of our relationship. It may be that when marriages are destroyed by a tragedy, the flaws in the relationship already existed. The way Tess helped her parents was to get on with life and her wide range of activities. She has done as much as anyone to rebuild our life together as a family. She has been a constant reminder that we need to move forward, that we still have our lives to live, that Jason would want us to enjoy whatever pleasures or challenges may come. Although Tess has been affected by Jason's death, she has used it to approach life with an appreciation far deeper than can be found in most adolescents.

As for professional life, I continued to function effectively in part because I believe in the importance of my work, but another critical factor was my deliberate and conscious involvement in the grieving process. American culture has a few brief rituals to facilitate the grieving process—public and private visitations, the funeral, the burial. All of them occur immediately after the death, and soon thereafter we are expected to resume our lives. Compared with many other cultures, ours does not provide an adequate grieving process for the difficult tasks of healing and achieving reconciliation with a death. Instead, each individual has to "invent" his or her own process, and mine involved the pursuit of activities that seemed to satisfy different needs.

Jan and I both believed that writing would help, and we each wrote regularly about our thoughts and feelings. We began by describing the scene at the hospital, but as we continued writing we moved in different directions. I described events in the present— the details of the funeral preparations, the private and public visitations, the funeral itself; but Jan wrote about the past, beginning with the last time she saw Jason and continuing to go backward in time. At one point she wrote what a college counselor had told her about Jason behaving like a role model during an orientation meeting for freshmen. While Jan searched her memories to recapture stories of the son we had lost, I was describing the experience of loss. When I began revising my journal writing into a manuscript, I thought about her stories and began including them and adding some of my own.

Although writing was essential for healing, I needed to do more. I wanted to do something for Jason, for his memory. I wanted to do something that would help me think of him and express my love for him. Jan primarily needed time to remember and revive the feelings from those memories. At work she often daydreamed, and at home she went through pictures and memorabilia, such as Jason's report cards from school, anything to help her remember and reconstruct a past that included Jason. When I recalled favorite memories of Jason, feelings of pain and loss would overwhelm me and I would weep. This made me feel helpless, so I needed to do things to give me a sense of control, a sense of purpose and meaning in response to this meaningless death. Writing helped, but I needed to do more, something to create the illusion of my son's presence.

I searched through Jason's writing. There was a small collection of poetry and prose in his papers. I was proud of his poems, especially those he wrote during his freshman year at college. In my favorite poem he writes of lying in bed at night in his dorm room, remembering his father reading to him every night. It is a poem written in words of love. So I used my computer to create a small anthology of his written work, and Jan designed a cover that included Jason's high school graduation picture. We printed the cover on a heavier stock of paper and produced 50 copies that we distributed to family and friends.

Another project was to use the $3,000 sent as donations by family and friends as the basis for establishing a scholarship fund in Jason's memory. Jan and I discussed this idea with a representative from a local foundation who said it would require a minimum of $15,000 to make enough interest from the fund to generate scholarships. We said we would make payments to the account in the coming years until we had accumulated that much money. This project provided a long-term goal, but I wanted to do something immediately to help me deal the pain.

To satisfy that need, I drafted a few letters to some of Jason's "heroes." He admired several people in the film industry including writers, directors, and even reviewers; but there were seven people who were especially significant to him. In the letters, I told them how much they had meant to him and thanked them for enriching his life. As I thought about mailing these letters, I was certain that the only way they would help me was if I took satisfaction simply from writing them. If I expected any of these celebrities to respond, I would probably be disappointed and hurt. I didn't need any more pain.

So I revised and sent these letters to the seven celebrities, sharing the story of my son's brief life and thanking them for having a positive influence on him. Each recipient was told that no response was necessary. Even so, three of the seven responded. George Lucas sent a signed poster, as did Steven Spielberg. Garrison Keillor did even more. He telephoned and talked to Jan, giving her his condolences, and during that conversation he offered to perform a benefit for Jason's scholarship fund. It was like a burst of light for two people struggling through the darkness of grief and despair.

I was also searching for books to read. I found some, and friends sent some, but most of them concerned terminal illness, so they offered little consolation. When people know they are dying, they have a chance to resolve things—heal old wounds, pay old debts, say goodbye to old friends and to the family. With an unexpected death, you are left with questions, ache for reasons; you try to make sense of a senseless event. So I reread my own journal, trying to be objective, and what I had written seemed like a good start for a manuscript. I continued writing regularly, but now I was writing for a possible audience. The structure that eventually emerged interspersed stories from Jason's life with a narrative that described my grief experience since his death. All of my various activities helped me, but the writing made it possible to manage my grief; it was a significant part of the healing that allowed me to function appropriately in my professional life.

Within a year I had completed the first draft of the book, and after several more years and numerous revisions, the book was published in 1994 as *The Fall of a Sparrow: Of Death and Dreams and Healing*. With this project concluded, it seemed that the "doing" phase of my grieving process was over. Although it was an inadequate substitute for having Jason with me, at least the story of his life was preserved. With this book I had given Jason a place in the world, a place he should have occupied as a living presence, but this would have to do.

I'm not sure where the next phase of my grief journey will take me, but healing takes a long time, perhaps a lifetime, and I will have to attend to it. Many things have helped, especially Garrison Keillor's benefit for Jason's scholarship fund. This benefit was such a significant event for my family, Jason's friends, and everyone who attended because it represented an affirmation of life and love and family. It affirmed Jason's place in my heart. It reminded us not to let our pain overwhelm our sense of joy. Since the accident I had often wondered if I could ever fully recapture my enthusiasm for life and work. At the benefit I heard Keillor saying that I could and that I should. I needed to hear that.

Perhaps the next phase of the grieving process may require a confrontation with the reality that a part of me died with Jason. I am not the person I was. That person had a son and a daughter. He loved them; he shared their hopes and fears, dreams and frustrations. Now he was a father with only one child. Although I will continue to love my daughter and participate in her life, it is not the same as before. There is an absence that has changed me, because the person I am now cannot forget the son who is no longer here. And that makes me a different person, not better or worse, just different.

Not only do I have to accept the death of my son, but also the death of the person I used to be. It is a hard thing to do. I liked the person I used to be and hope that the best parts of him will be maintained in the new person. Writing about my grief journey has been an important part of my healing, and I believe this writing has also made it possible to begin the next part of the journey.

According to a Buddhist proverb, "Life is joyful participation in the sorrows of the world." Perhaps these words should become part of the consciousness of this evolving person, this father who has lost a son and still cherishes his daughter. Perhaps this new person will contribute to the creation of a new family that now consists only of a father, mother, and daughter. The process is already happening, but I have not participated much in it. My wife and daughter have done most of the work. Writing the dedication for my book was the first time I had expressed my awareness of their efforts, but the words came almost effortlessly. These words are the proper ending for this essay:

> **To Jan and Tess**
> Who have loved
> amid the charred ruins of a family
> And created in the ashes
> like the phoenix
> A new family:
> smaller than before
> but just as beautiful.

REFERENCES

Millay, Edna St. Vincent. (1991). Dirge without music. In C. Falck (Ed.), *Selected poems*. New York: Perennial Classics.

Tennyson, Alfred. (1959). Break, break, break. In G. B. Harrison (Ed.), *Major British writers*. New York: Harcourt, Brace and World, Inc.

Wordsworth, William. (1936). Surprised by joy. In *Complete poetical works*, Oxford: Oxford University Press.

Yeats, W. B., Ego Dominus Tuus. In R. Finneran (Ed.), *The Yeats reader: A portable compendium of poetery, drama and prose* (p. 69). New York: Scribner Poetry. (Originally published in *The Wild Swans at Coole*, 1917.)

CHAPTER 2

Mortality:
A Matter of Life and Death

Faith, Sir, we are here today and gone tomorrow.
Mrs. Aphra Behn

Mrs. Behn exaggerates the brevity of life, and yet it is brief; a truth that is frequently ignored. People often speak of wanting to know "the truth" as if that will make them happy or empowered or liberated, and that believing in lies is wicked, vile, or at best naïve. Yet, acknowledging the fact that our all-too-brief lives ultimately end in death is to embrace a truth that feels more like a cactus than a comforter. It is not soothing; it would be better described as a bruising reality. The novelist Vladimir Nabokov (1999) expressed the truth about mortality as he saw it in the starkest terms: "Our existence is but a brief crack of light between two eternities of darkness" (p. 17).

Recognizing the possibility that death might mean the end of our consciousness and our existence can evolve into a fear of death that is overwhelming, paralyzing. If true, life can seem meaningless, and we may be tempted to ask, "what is the point of living?" And yet, most human beings appear to reject a nihilistic response to that question, and they go on with their lives. On what basis do we choose to live?

For many, the answer comes simply from faith—believing in God, in an immortal soul, and in promises of an afterlife. Further, visions of that afterlife may include options for the individual soul that may be determined by choices you make and actions you take during your lifetime. You may go to heaven or to purgatory or to hell. You may find yourself reincarnated as a Brahmin or as an untouchable. There is a complexity to all this that I am not addressing, but the main attraction of such predictions of an afterlife is a desire for justice that has been the basis of such beliefs for thousands of years. We have all seen the good people suffer harm while the wicked prosper, so if we cannot count on justice in this world, there must be another to make everything right.

> Death opens unknown doors.
> It is most grand to die.
> John Masefield

Kierkegaard said committing to any religion requires a leap of faith into the abyss. It is to believe in something that cannot be rationally proven. Theologians and people of faith have often tried to make religion as rational as possible, but in the end, all religious belief is irrational. It is irrational because the believer must accept truths with no clear and incontrovertible proof, based instead mostly on hearsay evidence (i.e., because of what is written in the Bible or the Qu'ran or another sacred text). The incontrovertible truth is that human beings are mortal. We know that each of us will die at some point despite developments in cryogenics, cloning, and the latest breakthrough in genome research. Technological innovations may prolong life, but not indefinitely.

What can a rational person do? One option is to accept the reality of death and to accommodate the prospect of a finite existence by making the most of the time you have. Many atheists operate this way, but atheism does not constitute a well-worn path. Some people choose an intellectual path, using their knowledge of human history and culture to tease out a rational basis for believing in God and in an immortal human spirit or soul. They learn how religions developed in cultures around the world and note the consistent patterns of belief in an immortal soul or spirit that survives the demise of the body. Many have argued that this widespread pattern is a compelling argument for the validity of such beliefs, but Mark Twain (1990) noted the weakness of such an argument: "One of the proofs of the immortality of the soul is that myriads have believed in it—they also believed the world was flat." Taking this intellectual approach is like walking into a minefield. No matter how skillfully a person negotiates the field, at some point he or she is likely to stumble on a perspective or a specific argument that seriously damages or destroys the beliefs that are guiding the sojourner on this difficult journey.

> We are made to be immortal, and yet we die.
> It's horrible; it can't be taken seriously.
> Eugene Ionesco

Another option some people choose is to assert that the human mind can never answer questions about whether immortality is possible, insisting that the human heart holds the answer. This believer follows a path guided by feelings more than intellect, especially feelings of love and compassion that create a sense of connection with others. Such believers may pursue a transcendental experience, believing that our spiritual selves will eventually merge into a mystical Oneness from which we came and to which we return. Some indigenous people have expressed such a belief and it is also part of the Jewish mystical tradition. Ralph Waldo Emerson borrowed such a belief to describe his concept of the "Oversoul." Spiritual beliefs often exist separate from the strictures of any particular religious ideology, and it may be comforting if the believer achieves a sense of being at peace with the world and with the brevity of time human beings have to live in it. Of course, it is not a universal truth but merely a belief, and like any belief it may turn out to be wrong.

> I warmed both hands before the fire of life;
> It sinks, and I am ready to depart.
> Walter Savage Landor

The well-worn path is the one people follow by identifying with a specific religious faith and accepting most beliefs associated with that faith. This ought to mean that the faithful will engage in behaviors consistent with their religious beliefs, but few people seem to be capable of consistently acting on religious principles in their daily lives. In response to such consistent inconsistency, many spiritual leaders contend that human beings are so deeply flawed that it is impossible for anyone to deserve the reward of heaven by good works, and that individual souls will be given permission to enter heaven only by the grace of God. And so on.

Despite whatever assurances they are given, human beings continue to search for a definitive answer to the question of whether we are merely mortal beings or if we possess an immortal soul. It is assumed that we will discover the answer when we die, but for most of us that is not soon enough. We want an answer that will fortify us before our confrontation with death, whenever that comes. In his book *The Tragic Sense of Life*, Miguel de Unamuno (1954) proposes an interesting hypothesis to resolve the ambiguities of human immortality. His concept of immortality was rooted in his concept of God:

> If there is a Universal and Supreme Consciousness, I am an idea in it; and is it possible for any idea in this Supreme Consciousness to be completely blotted out? After I have died, God will go on remembering me, and to be remembered by God, to have my consciousness sustained by the Supreme Consciousness, is not that, perhaps, to be? (p. 149)

To believe that each person is an idea in the mind of an immortal God is an appealing concept. It acknowledges each person's consciousness of being alive and connects each consciousness within a "Supreme Consciousness" that incorporates all people (past and present) into an unknowable omniscience. Unamuno's explanation combines intellectual and spiritual elements that blend into a mystical wholeness. Whether true or not, this argument offers a set of wings for those standing on the precipice, peering into that unfathomable abyss, preparing for the leap.

> Dying is a very dull, dreary affair.
> And my advice to you is to have
> nothing whatever to do with it.
> W. Somerset Maugham

Yet one problem with any belief in God is that such beliefs often include a belief in evil that some personify in the form of Satan or the devil. Some individuals may anguish over the immortality of their souls, while others imagine a cosmic contest between God and the devil to claim that soul. In response to the latter view, the poem included in this section is a shape poem. The persona of the poem is the devil and his comments appear in the shape of a question mark, a shape alluding to the questioning, doubting minds that make people vulnerable to visions of satanic forces at work. The question ending the poem paraphrases the ancient philosophical problem questioning the necessity for the existence of evil. For my part, I agree with a friend of mine who once said, "I believe it is antithetical to my spiritual health that I sometimes think there is a Hell."

The excerpts from wisdom literature pertaining to mortality in the boxed texts throughout this essay offer quite different, even contradictory perspectives. John Masefield argues that death represents a further exploration into unknown realms—a continuation of life's journey. Landors' comment suggests that death should simply be regarded as a fact of life, whereas Eugene Ionesco clearly perceives injustice if not tragedy in human mortality. Somerset Maugham injects a subtle levity into the topic, but he is serious in his insistence that there is nothing good about dying. British poet John Keats experienced illness and pain in his short life, and he expresses the sentiments of many in saying that for someone who is suffering, being dead is preferable to being alive because it offers the absence of pain.

> I have been half in love with easeful Death,
> Call'd him soft names in many a mused rhyme,
> To take into the air my quiet breath;
> Now more than ever seems it rich to die,
> To cease upon the midnight with no pain . . .
> John Keats

The one-act play concluding the chapter has the Angel of Death coming for a man who is not prepared to die, an idea inspired by a comment from French novelist Anatole France: "The average man, who does not know what to do with his life, wants another that will last forever." Ironically, *Lucky Man* was written on a rainy day when I could think of nothing to do. The idea was for death to have a dialogue with a man who had lived an "unexamined life," for him to realize what he has missed by treating the gift of life so casually, and yet to end in a way that allows him to be reconciled to his death.

his mark

a pitiful lack of truth;
in me   in sooth
You see   I'm odd,
a fraud!
The good,
they should
despise
my lies.
The wise
surmise,
but those
disposed
to sin
begin
to stray
away;
'tis these
(with ease)
I take
to bake
and burn.
I yearn,
and roar
for more!

'tis fit . . .
ain't it?

LUCKY MAN

Adam Mensch—a man in his 50s
Death—an angel of death

Scene: A television set facing away from the audience, an easy chair faces the television. Adam sits in the easy chair watching television, but there is no sound. Dim stage lighting, the audience can see Adam in the glow from the television.

Offstage Voice: The average man, who does not know what to do with his life, wants another that will last forever.

(*Death enters and the stage lights go up.*)

    DEATH
Adam Mensch?

    ADAM
What?

    DEATH
It's me. I've come.

    ADAM
Who are you? What are you talking about?

    DEATH
You're going to die now and come with me.

    ADAM
What? Now? Wait. Now?

    DEATH
Yes.

    ADAM
Wait. What? Hold on. Why me?

    DEATH
It's time.

    ADAM
Now?

DEATH
Now.

ADAM
Wait. You're kidding, right?

DEATH
Look at me.

ADAM
You're serious.

DEATH
Dead serious.

ADAM
Come on now . . . Who are you? Really.

DEATH
I've told you. Please come with me now. It's time.

ADAM
Wait. I can't . . . I'm not ready.

DEATH
That makes no difference to me.

ADAM
It makes a difference to me! I'm not ready.

DEATH
All right. I'm a little early. I have some time to kill. Just for the sake of hesitation, why aren't you ready?

ADAM
Because . . . I'm . . . I still . . . enjoy . . . things.

DEATH
Things.

ADAM
Sunrises, rainbows, the sounds of children playing . . . smelling cinnamon rolls, sipping a glass of wine. Red wine. Holding my wife's hand . . . walking . . . standing. I like standing. So, see?

DEATH
I see that you've covered all five senses, very clever.

ADAM
Yes, all five, and I'm not tired of any of them yet. The cup isn't half full; it's half empty. There, I've solved that little conundrum for you.

DEATH
A conundrum for you perhaps, not for me.

ADAM
Okay, fine, but you see my point. I need more time . . . to fill the cup. When my cup "runneth over," then you can come for me.

DEATH
I see your point, and it may surprise you to learn that others have made this point, but it's irrelevant. Do you understand why?

ADAM
Right now? No, no I don't understand. Let me think about it.

DEATH
You do not get to determine when you die.

ADAM
But some people do. The last year before he died, my Uncle was in pain every day. He couldn't get out of bed. He had to wear diapers. He was humiliated. He prayed for death to come.

DEATH
Yes, I remember. He came quite willingly.

ADAM
Well, I'm not suffering like that. I'm not, and I'm not ready to go. I mean, I have a few aches and pains, stairs can be difficult, but I'm not ready to throw in the towel.

DEATH
Throw in the towel? You talk as though life were a boxing match.

ADAM
It is! I mean, it's sort of like a boxing match. But it's fixed! Every one of us is going to kiss the canvas sometime. Death always wins. But I want to go all 15 rounds. I'm still standing. I enjoy standing.

DEATH
Why?

ADAM
To stay alive! I want to go on living.

DEATH
That's such an adolescent attitude. Teenagers think they are immortal. It's always a big shock when I show up. They become weepy and are full of regret, but you're an adult! I expect a more mature response from an adult. In fact, I insist upon it. At this point in your life you should know that it's inevitable. You should be prepared for Death. It should make no difference whether it's today or tomorrow.

ADAM
It makes a lot of difference! Okay? I mean . . . I don't understand this whole thing . . . I need time . . . I don't just mean dying. I mean life! I'm still trying to figure out life. If I understood that, then, you know, dying might not be so bad. I would . . . I would probably be ready to go or something, but I mean, come on. I still don't know if God exists, and that makes it difficult for me to have, you know, religious beliefs . . . which would probably help me, right now. I have questions . . . a lot of questions. And it would help to have, you know, answers . . . I need answers

DEATH
Why?

ADAM
Well, if I had some answers . . . to things . . . I could, maybe I could be reconciled, a little, to my fate, and then maybe I could go with you. But I mean, don't you see? I have questions.

DEATH
Perhaps I should give you answers and let you tell me what the question is. You want Death to be a game show host who explains things you don't understand. You couldn't do it on your own, so now you want a short cut? Sorry, I don't answer questions. I'm just an escort.

ADAM
I didn't call for your services.

DEATH
You can't be too frightened if you can make such bad jokes.

ADAM
Everyone's a critic . . . you could just laugh, you know.

DEATH
Don't take offence; I never laugh. It's not appropriate.

ADAM
Why?

DEATH
Because laughter is a sign of camaraderie and friendship; the rules are very strict about getting too close to the clients.

ADAM
I thought you were supposed to accept me.

DEATH
I do accept you, but I don't have to like you.

ADAM
What did I do?

DEATH
That is a relevant question, isn't it?

ADAM
What?

DEATH
What did you ever do in your entire life that might make anyone like or dislike you?

ADAM
Wait. What?

DEATH
Never mind, but I do have opinions about people. Gandhi, for example, was a lovely man. Great conversations. Albert Schweitzer was a bit esoteric for my taste, all that "reverence for life" business, but Eleanor Roosevelt? Fascinating. And Martin Luther King gave me such a hug when we met, delightful man.

ADAM
So you're responsible for "escorting" everyone? Aren't you incredibly busy?

DEATH
There are many escorts; you're all covered. But fate, or perhaps fortune, has allowed me to be the companion for some very special people.

ADAM
So which people were you not so crazy about?

DEATH
Quite a few, but you wouldn't know them. Obviously the names I've already mentioned are well known. I could have mentioned Ralph Wilson, Juanita Perez, Mustafa Ali, or Mia Yang. I know you don't recognize those names, but they were all good, kind, and decent people, helpful to others, even strangers. They made their communities better, and when it was their turn to go they were mature about it and went willingly.

ADAM
I'm mature . . . I'm mature!

DEATH
It goes without saying.

ADAM
Then stop bringing it up! But c'mon, weren't there some people you didn't like?

DEATH
I could mention some famous people you would recognize, but I'd rather not. No point in speaking ill of the dead. There are many people I have not enjoyed escorting: remorseless criminals, greedy CEOs, psychopaths, dentists . . .

ADAM
Okay, sure, I can see that.

DEATH
I was joking about the dentists. I wanted to see if you were paying attention—obviously you were not.

ADAM
So you can tell jokes?

DEATH
Well, I mostly do sight gags, but yes, sometimes I joke. But I never laugh.

ADAM
Are you serious?

DEATH
No, I'm Death.

ADAM
Ha, ha. But really, I'm interested. How about a couple of names of people you didn't like.

DEATH
No, but I will do this: I'll set the record straight on a few famous people who have been misrepresented. Brutus, Cassius, and Judas were not the most evil people who ever lived, trapped forever in the mouth of Satan and agonizingly masticated.

ADAM
Umm, is that from Dante's Inferno?

DEATH
Very good. Dante's love of Caesar blinded him. Brutus was a noble and generous soul, a bit boring but a good man. Cassius was a great talker—passionate, principled, animated. He was wonderful company. And Judas, Judas was simply a well-intentioned boob. He didn't betray Jesus; he simply played the part he was supposed to play. As you say in America, "No harm, no foul."

ADAM
No harm, no foul! He got Jesus crucified!

DEATH
That was going to happen regardless. Someone had to make it possible, and Judas happened to be the one. Later he regretted it. He was full of remorse. Such despair. So you see, he was quite a moral person, and he behaved like a mature adult ought to behave.

ADAM
Would you stop already with the mature stuff?

DEATH
Fine. As long as you start acting mature and come with me. Now.

ADAM
Wait, wait just a minute. I'm confused by what you're saying about Judas; it sounds like you're talking about predestination. Are you saying every person's fate is determined and we have no free will?

DEATH
Of course you have free will; you have no choice.

ADAM
Another one of your jokes?

DEATH
Actually, it's not mine; I borrowed it from a Jewish writer. It's more of a paradox really, or as William Blake used to say, a "contrary." Look, you don't have any choice about being free to choose. Romeo could babble on about the stars dictating his destiny, but Shakespeare knew the truth; that's why he gave those lines to a confused adolescent. All humanity has the ability to make choices for which there are consequences, and "What's done cannot be undone."

ADAM
You're quoting literature here, but this is a religious issue.

DEATH
Literature. Religion. Secular. Sacred. Potato. Potahto.

ADAM
So what are you saying, that nothing is sacred?

DEATH
That is so typical, so American. Is nothing sacred? Please. Everything is sacred. You might have understood that if Americans had paid attention to Indians instead of trying to annihilate them, in the name of God, of course.

ADAM
I think we're getting off track here. We were talking about free will. Can we get back to that?

DEATH
If that's your choice.

ADAM
Maybe it's not my choice. Listen: if god is omniscient then he knows everything that has happened, is happening and will happen. So, how can anyone make a real choice? That choice has already been made in the mind of god; nothing can be done to change it.

DEATH
So, you want to play these silly little games of logic?

ADAM
I'm just saying . . .

DEATH
Fine, but understand this, when you use human logic you are bound by the limitations of the human mind. Does predestination make sense if god is not only omniscient but also omnipotent?

ADAM
Wait. What?

DEATH
If god is all-knowing and all-powerful, then god can do whatever god wants. If god doesn't want to know what choices human beings are going to make, god can choose not to know.

ADAM
But . . . how . . .

DEATH
If there is a god.

ADAM
If?

DEATH
I'm just saying . . .

ADAM
See, this is hard.

DEATH
Not so hard. People who think this way are just trying to use logic to avoid the consequences for their actions.

ADAM
Meaning?

DEATH
They want god to be responsible for everything. People actually like the idea of a devil because if there is a devil then god created him (or her) and is responsible for whatever mischief the devil does. When people give in to temptation they simply say, "The devil made me do it." That makes it god's fault and they get to act as if they're not responsible.

ADAM
So what? It's true isn't it? God has to be responsible.

DEATH
It's a con game that humans play upon themselves (*oratorical flourish*), but when the smoke of all this obfuscation is blown away by the winds of truth . . . ah, excuse me, I'm sorry . . . But the truth is that at the end of the day, what you find is that a human being has the freedom to make good choices or bad ones.

ADAM
Okay, so I have free will. Okay, fine, then I choose not to leave with you.

DEATH
You can be amusing even though you do not seem very bright. There are limits to free will, the primary one being mortality. You have free will while you are alive, but when you . . . when your escort arrives, you no longer have free will, no control over what happens.

ADAM
See, that's the problem. That's the real problem with this "journey" you want me to take. I don't know where the path goes or what's at the end of it. If I knew more about that, I might be, you know, more willing to leave.

DEATH
What about your love of life? The half-full cup?

ADAM
Okay look, just between you and me, I know that the best years of my life are behind me.

DEATH
Oh really? You already knew that?

ADAM
Most of the good stuff in my life is a repetition of past experiences, and it's never as good as the first time . . . I mean, it's still good . . . but . . . okay, take sex.

DEATH
I'm not that kind of escort.

ADAM
Oh, you are funny. Have a little respect, okay? We're talking about my life here. So, anyway, when two people are attracted to each other and have sex, it's a great experience. I mean, you're making love and suddenly you are as physically close to another human being as you can be. There's passion. Excitement. Fireworks! But after a hundred or a thousand times, you know, it's sort of like a bottle rocket. Sparks, sure, but not, you know, Kaboom!

DEATH
After a thousand times?

ADAM
Give or take.

DEATH
So, let's see if I understand what you're saying. You're ready to leave because your sex life doesn't kaboom?

ADAM
No, no, no! C'mon, I'm trying to explain here. I'm just saying I might be persuaded to, you know, go . . . with you, but I need to know what's going to happen after I die. This long journey—what's that about?

DEATH
I am not permitted to talk about that.

ADAM
Who says? Who won't let you talk?

DEATH
I am not permitted to talk . . .

ADAM
Aha! You see? That's my problem.

DEATH
But it's not my problem.

ADAM
Look, could you at least tell me if there is a god and what god is like? That would help a lot. And while you're at it, what about religion, you know, which one got it right?

DEATH
I can answer that question—none of them.

ADAM
No religion understands god? But . . . wait . . . not even . . . why not? Because there is no god, is that it?

DEATH
What I'm saying is that none of them understands the true nature of eternity. They don't accurately explain what happens when you die, and frankly most of them have made a mess of telling people how to live. A wise man once said, "We have just enough religion to make us hate, but not enough to make us love one another." Religion has been one of the major causes of suffering and death.

ADAM
What about . . .

DEATH
No, not even them.

ADAM
What about . . .

DEATH
Oh please, don't even start. Human beings have simply missed the mark when it comes to religion.

ADAM
If we had got it right, what would we be doing?

DEATH
I am not permitted to talk about that.

ADAM
And what if I choose to know more about that?

DEATH
Then we will have much to talk about on the journey.

ADAM
So, you'll tell me the meaning of life and what god is like and, you know, all that?

DEATH
As long as you are interested.

ADAM
But how about now? Before we leave, anything?

DEATH
No. To be alive is to be mortal, partial, limited. Haven't you read the Bible? There is that wonderful comment that to be alive is to "see through the glass darkly," but once you are dead, you will come "face to face" with the truth.

ADAM
Learning by dying.

DEATH
Yes. You will see what you could not see and know what was not known.

ADAM
That sounds like we're immortal? Are we? Do I have an immortal soul?

DEATH
I didn't say that.

ADAM
So what are you saying? That we find out everything and then disappear into nothingness? That's absurd! What is the point of that?

DEATH
I can say nothin . . .

ADAM
But can't you just . . .

DEATH
Nothing. (Adam starts to speak) Nothing. Don't you understand?

ADAM
And if I said no?

DEATH
Then I'll say I'm sorry but I can say no more.

ADAM
Okay, you're right. I do have a problem. Look, I need to understand what this "journey" of yours is about; I need to know where I'm going.

DEATH
You must leave this life knowing nothing.

ADAM
There you go again; look, that's what bothers me. Not only that I know nothing, but that I might become nothing. You know? It's like that poem I had to read in college—"When I Have Fears That I May Cease To Be." Those fears. That's what haunts me.

DEATH
Meaning?

ADAM
Sometimes when I go to bed, I get restless, can't sleep. I start thinking . . . you know, about dying. Not dying really, but being . . . dead. I really have a hard time believing in a god, or heaven and hell and all that, you know. It just seems like a fantasy. Logic tells me we just become nothing. No more consciousness, no more joy or pain. Oblivion.

DEATH
And this bothers you?

ADAM
I hate it!

DEATH
Why?

ADAM
Because . . . I mean . . . I don't know . . . I just don't know! But if it all comes to nothing then, I mean, it makes me anxious; I get afraid. Some nights these fears seem to be strangling me and I can't stop from moaning and tossing and turning. Then I have to get up because . . . I just have to. I want to sleep . . . but I can't.

DEATH
Have you tried counting sheep?

ADAM
It makes me think of lambs going to the slaughter. Sometimes . . . I almost hope there is a hell . . . because feeling pain seems better than not existing, being nothing.

DEATH
Six of one, half a dozen of the other. Are you sure you would prefer pain?

ADAM
I'm not sure of anything. When my Uncle was dying, there was so much pain, he begged for you. He prayed for you to come. And he wasn't very religious.

DEATH
Ah, religion. Pray not to die; pray to die; pray not to have pain; pray to have pain so that you know you're alive. God knows what people want.

ADAM
Aha, so there is a God!

DEATH
It's just an expression.

ADAM
Okay fine, but tell me this, why did my Uncle have to suffer so long? Where were you? Why didn't you come and get him?

DEATH
You should read more Stephen Crane.

ADAM
What? I mean . . . I would, if I had more time.

DEATH
Just listen:
A man said to the universe:
"Sir, I exist!"
"However," replied the universe,
"The fact has not created in me
A sense of obligation."

ADAM
That's Stephen Crane?

DEATH
That's Stephen Crane.

ADAM
And that helps me how?

DEATH
Look, I'm getting tired of this. It's time to go.

ADAM
Okay. Just wait a sec . . . I'll go, okay, and I'll even go quietly, under one condition.

DEATH
Condition? I am Death. You can't bargain . . .

ADAM
Just hear me out. Please. Wouldn't you prefer that I came along willingly? I'm just trying to come up with a "win/win" solution here.

DEATH
A win/win solution? You're arguing with Death you idiot! . . . I'm sorry. Excuse me. . . All right, so tell me, what do you need to "win?"

ADAM
I just want to know if I become something after I die. I'm not asking you to tell me what. I'm not asking if there's a heaven or hell or Nirvana or any of that. You don't have to tell me if I will remember who I was. I can accept the loss of my personality; hell, I insist! I could accept the idea that I become part of some life force, a World Soul or something. But I want to know if some part of me survives, and if that

part might return to earth. Is reincarnation . . . I mean, I just want to know . . . I'd like . . . Don't get me wrong; I don't mean to insist . . .

DEATH
Oh no, you wouldn't want to start being pushy now . . .

ADAM
I'm sorry. When I get anxious or nervous, I talk. I ramble.

DEATH
Obviously. Before I respond, I have a question for you. If eternity is a state of perpetual bliss as some humans believe, would you still prefer coming back to earth where there is so much suffering?

ADAM
I don't know. I don't know what perpetual bliss is like.

DEATH
But you have some idea. Sex is apparently a kind of bliss and they say ignorance is bliss—you certainly have your share of that. So, how about it? If you had a choice, would you choose coming back to earth or "eternal bliss?"

ADAM
Do I have a choice? I thought you said I didn't have a choice.

DEATH
I'm just curious about your preference.

ADAM
What about this? I've often wondered if eternity might be determined by what a person believes it is going to be. You know; what you think is what you get?

DEATH
I'm asking the questions now. Which option would you prefer?

ADAM
I don't know if I have a preference. I like the idea of coming back to earth as someone else, especially if I can have memories of my former lives like people talk about when they're hypnotized. I mean, is that stuff for real or what?

DEATH
I wish you would stop trying to trick me into answering questions I am not allowed to answer.

ADAM
Okay, you can't tell me. But reincarnation would probably be my choice, mainly because I kind of know about that. I don't know what eternal bliss is like. I know temporary bliss, but I can't imagine stretching that out over eternity. Wouldn't that get boring?

DEATH
So, given a choice, you would prefer to come back to earth.

ADAM
Well, as a human. I mean, I wouldn't want to come back as a bat or a bug, you know, like a mayfly; they only live 24 hours to mate and die. They don't even have a digestive track. Did you know that?

DEATH
I don't do mayflies.

ADAM
Okay, I'm just saying that I enjoy, you know, sex, but it hardly seems worth it to come back for only 24 hours, even if you get to screw your brains out.

DEATH
Oh, do mayflies have brains?

ADAM
I don't know. Look, my point is, if I come back to earth, I want to come back as a conscious being who can appreciate life.

DEATH
That was your option this time. How did that work out for you?

ADAM
Are you trying to be funny?

DEATH
Apparently you don't think so. Anyway, you would choose to be human again. But what if you came back as an impoverished child living

on the streets of Bombay or Sao Paulo or Chicago? Would you still choose to be reincarnated?

ADAM
I don't know. It doesn't make sense to come back to earth if you're just going to suffer. What kind of life is that? What's the point of living if all you feel is pain?

DEATH
Yet earlier you said you would prefer suffering to death, just as long as you were conscious of being alive.

ADAM
Well, as long as there's some way to get away from the suffering.

DEATH
And if you couldn't? Would that be so bad? Dostoyevsky said suffering was good for the soul.

ADAM
Then let him suffer, but leave me out of it. That's why I never read those Russian writers; I heard they were gloomy, going on and on about suffering and death, you know, kind of obsessed with that stuff.

DEATH
Ah Mr. Sunshine, you think they were too gloomy . . .

ADAM
I'm not obsessed with mortality! I am worried about nonexistence, about becoming nothing. I thought I had made that clear.

DEATH
Yes, as clear as a looking glass.

ADAM
I'm serious!

DEATH
And I'm Death. And this has gone on far too long. It's time to leave.

ADAM
I'm still not ready. Just wait . . .

DEATH
It doesn't matter if you're ready or not. (*reaches for Adam's arm*)

ADAM
(*pulls his arm away*) So it's "ready or not, here I come?" Shouldn't I get to hide first? Shouldn't you have to find me? Why should this be easy for you and hard for me?

DEATH
You're stalling. And your time is up. (*holds out his hand.*)

ADAM
Wait. No. I'm not stalling. I am not stalling. Why would I stall? (*Death grabs Adam's shoulder*) Hey, you're hurting me.

DEATH
Don't worry; the pain is temporary. (*Adam steps backward but Death maintains his grip*) It will only hurt more, the more you resist.

ADAM
Wait. Wait! (*in pain, Adam falls on one knee and weeps*)

DEATH
Stop that! Stop that right now! Look, I don't know how else to tell you. You have no choice. You must come with me. I can't tell you what happens next because you're not supposed to know.

ADAM
I know . . . But . . . Okay, how about this. Can you just tell me . . . if anybody came close to understanding what happens after we die? That wouldn't be telling me too much, would it? I'm not asking you to tell me what's on the other side of the glass. Just tell me this: Did any human being ever come up with something that came close to the truth?

DEATH
Then will you come with me, quietly?

ADAM
(*Adam rises*) Yes, I promise.

DEATH
When I tell you, you can't say it's not enough. You can't say you need something more. I'll tell you and then we must go. No more stalling.

ADAM
Stalling? Me? I'm not . . . Okay, I just need a shred of truth, something to help me be, you know, not so afraid.

DEATH
One person came close, quite close, actually. Walt Whitman. *Leaves of Grass*. Have you read it?

ADAM
Yes. Well, some of it anyway.

DEATH
Do you remember this?
All goes onward and outward, nothing collapses,
And to die is different from what any one supposed, and luckier.

ADAM
That's it?

DEATH
That's as close as it comes.

ADAM
Luckier? . . . Luckier?

DEATH
Now we must go.

ADAM
To be honest, I still don't want to . . . But I know I have no choice.

DEATH
Now you are being ma . . .

ADAM
Do I?

DEATH
Do I really have to answer that?

ADAM
I guess not, but listen, I've got a quote for you.

DEATH
Come on; you're just stalling for time and your time is up.

ADAM
I'm not stalling; I mean it. I just want you to know how I'm feeling.

DEATH
All right. What is it?

ADAM
Somebody said something like this: I don't mind dying; I just don't want to be there when it happens.

DEATH
(*smiles, covers his mouth with his hand*)

ADAM
Made you laugh. I made Death laugh.

DEATH
No you didn't; it was Woody Allen.

ADAM
What?

DEATH
It was Woody Allen who said it. And anyway, I wasn't laughing, I was just smiling. (*offers his arm*)

ADAM
And it's okay to smile? (*takes Death's arm and immediately waves his free hand by his head*) What's that?

DEATH
It's just a fly.

ADAM
I'm going to miss that.

DEATH
The buzzing of a fly?

ADAM
Yeah, I'm going to miss all of it.

DEATH
Well, all right, good for you.

ADAM
You're smiling again. So you can smile but not laugh. (*Death turns to leave but Adam doesn't move, loses contact with Death's arm*) What other rules do you have to follow? (*Death stops, turns*) By the way, how do you get to be an escort anyway? You know, I really think that's something I could do. (*Death shakes his head*) Hey, I'm serious here.

DEATH
And I am Death. (*holds out his arm*)

ADAM
I'm sorry to tell you this, but it wasn't funny the first time. But really, how do you become an escort? Is there an application process? Who does the interviews? Oh my god! Do you interview with . . . ? (*Adam takes Death's arm and they begin walking*) That reminds me, I've got a lot of questions, so I might as well start getting some answers. But don't let me forget about that escort thing. I want to come back to that, okay? But let's start with the big one. So tell me, is there a God?

(*As they leave the stage the lights dim and we can once again see the glow of the television set illuminating the empty chair*)

QUOTATIONS/REFERENCES NOT ATTRIBUTED IN THE TEXT

The average man, who does not know what to do with his life, wants another that will last forever.
>Anatole France
>(French author, 1844–1924)

Of course we have free will, we have no choice.
>Isaac Bashevis Singer
>(Jewish author, 1904–1991)

What's done cannot be undone.
>William Shakespeare (Macbeth)
>(English poet/playwright, 1564–1616)

We have just enough religion to make us hate, but not enough to make us love one another.
>Jonathan Swift
>(English author, 1667–1745)

When I have fears that I may cease to be
          John Keats
          (English poet, 1796–1821)

I heard a fly buzz when I died
          Emily Dickinson
          (American poet, 1830–1886)

REFERENCES

Behn, Aphra, (1995). The lucky chance. In M. Summers (Ed.), *The works of Aphra Behn* (Vol. III). Columbus: Ohio State University. http://onlinebooks.library.upenn.edu (by title or author).
France, Anatole. www.worldofquotes.com/author/Anatole-France.
Nabokov, Vladimir. (1999). *Speak, Memory*. New York: Everyman Library.
Twain, Mark. (1900). *Notebook*. www.twainquotes.com/Immortality.html
Unamuno, Miguel de. 1954). *Tragic sense of life*. New York: Dover Publications.

PART 2

Responding to an Unexpected Death

Some, too fragile for winter winds,
The thoughtful grave encloses,–
Tenderly tucking them in from frost
Before their feet are cold.

Never the treasures in her nest
The cautious grave exposes,
Building where schoolboy dare not look
And sportsman is not bold.

This covert have all the children
Early aged, and often cold,–
Sparrows unnoticed by the Father;
Lambs for whom time had not a fold.
                    Emily Dickinson (1959, p. 45)

CHAPTER 3

Bereavement: Becoming a Survivor

> *The fairest things have fleetest end,*
> *Their scent survives their close;*
> *But the rose's scent is bitterness*
> *To him that loved the rose.*
>   Francis Thompson (1919, p. 1)

A day or two after my son's death I found his bathrobe, and I held it to my face to breathe in the smell. I did this often for the next few days until his smell dissipated from the cloth. It was the sour scent of sweat, but it smelled sweet to me. I was despondent when the scent was gone, but the absence of Jason's smell reinforced the reality of his physical absence. My son was gone, forever. I could delay no longer. I had to begin the journey of learning how to get on with my life—to do what had to be done to become a "survivor." Others were already on this journey, and some were among people I knew—in some cases the parents had lost their child so long ago that no one talked about it any more, and for that reason I had not been aware of their loss.

I have approached many people to talk about their grief journey, especially parents who lost a child—hoping to learn from them by listening to their advice on how to grieve and to share the choices and actions that have helped me. After just a few conversations, it was apparent that even though the pain is similar, everyone grieves differently. One's memories of a child who dies are like rocks strewn across the path of your grief journey, and when you stumble upon them they stir up images. Some of the images are nostalgic, pleasant, yet they inevitably remind you of your child's absence. For me, it was worth the pain to remember the past, but this was not true for everyone.

> I have often wondered for what good end
> the sensations of Grief could be intended.
> Thomas Jefferson

About a year after my son died, I read in the newspaper that a former neighbor of mine had lost her only child in a car accident; her daughter was almost the same age as Jason when he died. Two years passed before I happened to see her at a restaurant and spoke to her. After a few minutes of conversation, I asked how she was feeling and followed by asking specifically how she had dealt with the loss of her daughter. She said, "I never think about it," and immediately steered the conversation to another topic. Did her comment mean that not only did she not think about the loss of her only child but that her daughter's death was so painful she did not allow herself to remember what they had done during the time they had been together?

There are many ways to deal with grief, and it is absurd to think that there are right ways or wrong ways to grieve. Even so, I struggled to understand how this mother's refusal to think about her daughter could constitute an effective way to resolve her grief. Wouldn't it require an extraordinary amount of psychic energy to blot out the reality that was your child's life? How does not thinking about a child who has died address the void that this absence creates in your life? I feel Jason's absence every day, so when I recall memories of him, it is like resurrecting his spirit. He comes alive for me again—if only in my mind, if only for a moment. Despite the pain that comes with remembering, not to remember Jason would be to confine him to the darkness of the grave. Recollections may cause pain, but they can also offer a joy that nourishes. As I have traveled the difficult and sometimes treacherous path of this grief journey, I have frequently stumbled over memories of Jason, but I have learned not to fall into despair.

> Between grief and nothing,
> I will take grief.
> William Faulkner

To lose a child is to lose your hopes and dreams for that child, and that loss can provoke profound despair. Reeling from the pain of losing a child, some people can seem almost suicidal, and their words of despair echo Emile Cioran's comment: "Since all life is futility, the decision to exist must be the most irrational of all." For a parent to bury a child defies rationality, contradicting reasonable human expectations and a basic sense of justice. At Jason's funeral, my father said,

"I should have been the one who died," and Jason's other grandfather made the same comment. It is hard to accept the randomness in life, especially when such events make no sense, serve no purpose. Yet it also serves no purpose to get caught up in the maelstrom of such thoughts. They lead nowhere, except perhaps to an obsession with one's own pain, oblivious to the pain of others.

Thomas Jefferson doubted that grief brought one to a "good end," but one of the purposes of grief is to remind us that we are not alone, that we have not been singled out for divine punishment. Other family members feel pain; other families have survived this kind of loss. The parents learn to comfort their other children; spouses learn to comfort each other. And in surviving, they may be comforted by family and friends or even neighbors. People send cards and flowers; people bring food to your home. They are expressing affection and a compassion, perhaps too seldom expressed, and it is all the more precious for being rarely experienced.

> A man's dying is more the
> survivor's affair than his own.
> Thomas Mann

According to obituaries, people who die are "survived by" a list of those who loved them. As human beings we have limited power. Some problems are easily solved, but we cannot fix every problem that disrupts our lives. For the ones that can't be resolved, we must do what we can to make our lives as meaningful and as satisfying as possible. We do this for ourselves and for others—whether at home or at work or in the community. We can minimize the damage of a loss by continuing to be part of a family and a community, and this is critical for making the transition to being "a survivor."

Some people deal with a loss by spending more time at the workplace, and for a time I pursued that path. Being at work provided a focus, pushing grief into the background. At work I could go for hours without a conscious thought of Jason, but as I drove home from work, a song might come on the radio that would remind me of him, and the tears would flow freely. So I let them. Driving around in the privacy of my car, I allowed my grief to take over, knowing that it would gradually diminish. When the pain eased, I would drive home, park the car in my garage and walk into my home, prepared to be the husband and father and friend that my family needed.

Grief does not simply wash over you like a wave with no lasting effect, but it does ebb and flow. It can come at any time—while reading, listening to music, or watching television. The anguish we feel often comes from never finding a good answer for the insistent question about why our loved one had to die.

> Why should a dog, a horse, a rat, have life,
> And thou no breath at all? Thou'lt come no more,
> Never, never, never, never, never!
> William Shakespeare

When it is especially painful, some people turn to alcohol to numb the pain, but the relief that alcohol provides comes at too high a price with little genuine benefit. Even the "blessing" of sleep induced by alcohol does not nurture one's mind and body like a normal night's sleep. For years I had enjoyed beer or wine on weekends, but as I note in the essay for this chapter, my desire to numb the pain led to drinking on nights during the week. One consequence was that I gained a lot of weight before finally forcing myself to acknowledge that alcohol was not good for one's physical, mental, or spiritual health. I knew that it could destroy marriages and ruin lives, so before allowing it to become that destructive in my life, I stopped using alcohol to ease my pain.

As I write this, my grief journey is approaching its 19th year, as many years as my son lived. I have learned how to be a survivor, but there is no road map others could follow because each individual's journey is different. My only advice is that you have to respond to the loss by finding a way to be hopeful, that this is not only necessary for you but for your family. That sentiment first surfaced in a poem called "Survival," written during the early stages of my grief journey. Parents who lose a child are often mired in guilt, regret, and despair, not perceiving any hope to comfort them. Surviving requires some form of hope. It may be a hope that your child is in a better place, in an afterlife where you will see him or her again. Others may find hope in the lives of their remaining children, a hope that their lives will be long and joyful. Others may become actively engaged in a cause related to the child they have lost, hoping for success to honor the memory of that child. Being comforted by some kind of hope can provide a way to accept that child's death. Although the poem ends without a resolution, it affirms our human need to be "hope-full."

> There is no flock, however watched and tended,
> But one dead lamb is there!
> There is no fireside, howsoe'er defended
> But has one vacant chair!
> Henry Wadsworth Longfellow

The excerpts from wisdom literature included in this chapter relate to bereavement, and many address the feeling of hopelessness that must be overcome. Thomas Jefferson's wife died at 33 years of age, less than 4 months after the birth of their fourth child. Because his grief did not ease his suffering, Jefferson cannot imagine a possible purpose for grief. William Faulkner refutes Jefferson by arguing that if the alternative to grief means feeling nothing at the loss of a loved one, he would prefer to grieve. Thomas Mann reminds us that no one else can tell us how to live with the loss of a loved one; it is a journey we must make on our own. Shakespeare's King Lear rages against the injustice that his beloved daughter Cordelia is dead while lesser beings are still alive; but Henry Wadsworth Longfellow counters Lear's emphasis on his individual suffering by offering survivors the assurance that all of us are survivors, that we are part of a community of grief and should not feel alone as we struggle with our loss.

The essay that concludes this chapter was written 8 years after my son died. Even though 8 years may seem like a long time, survivors will tell you that it is a brief period in a grief journey. "The Dance of Grief" describes choices my wife and I made as we grieved our son's death. During such a journey, each of us has to make certain choices, and many would probably not make the same choices that Jan and I made, but most of the activities we chose to do were right for us. This essay primarily emphasizes that people who are grieving must do whatever they believe will help them, no matter what others may think. Becoming a survivor means doing things that allow you or your family to go forward, not to become mired in guilt or pity but to keep moving ahead. The journey may seem endless, but like any journey there is much to gain simply by progressing along the path that stretches out before us.

SURVIVAL

Stomping his shoes, a shadowy hope
Beat thunderously on my front door.
    "Nobody home!" I shout.
But the persistent pounding
Forced me from the kitchen chair
Where I sat buttering my bread.

"Stop that," I say.
    "I can't use what you're selling."
"Too bad," says a voice,
    then footsteps fade away.
I wait a while, but the unwanted guest is gone.
Turning toward the kitchen, I seem to see
A small shadow slipping out the back door
    onto the dark porch,
A blur dashing past a circle of light;
    a screen door slams
    to confirm the intrusion.

I cannot find my slice of bread
    and the butter knife is gone.

I still feel hungry,
    but I leave the comfortable kitchen,
    to stand inside that circle of light.
Staring into the darkness,
    I imagine myself
    eating bread.

THE DANCE OF GRIEF

*Except for the point, the still point,
There would be no dance, and there is only the dance.*
T. S. Eliot (1967, p. 1309)

It is only a few weeks until my birthday. I will be 50 years old. My daughter will call to wish me a "Happy Birthday," and that will cause me to think about my son. Had he lived, Jason would be 27. I often speculate on what his life would be like if he were still alive. I cannot bear to think such thoughts on his birthday in July nor on the day he died in September. I resist such thoughts on those occasions because they would be too painful, but on my birthday, I like to remember the son who should be here with me or who would have called me like his sister to celebrate his father's birthday.

It has been more than 8 years since the accident. For the first few years I would occasionally drive over the bridge that crosses the Mississippi River and make my way to the winding road where he lost his life. I would stop and stare at the ditch that cradled him in its long grass, then kneel down on the soil that soaked up his blood, hoping to feel a sense of his presence. Afterwards I would drive on to the television station where he worked, turn around, and drive back on the last stretch of road he ever saw. Coming upon the turn in the road where Jason drove onto the shoulder, I could never understand why, but the logic of what happened next is tragically transparent. The first few times I returned, the gouged earth and debris were still there, but eventually tall grass hid the gouges, shattered glass and the rest. Nature does not work so quickly on the human heart.

I am better now than I was.

I have had help from family and friends, from dreams and the drama and drudgery of everyday life. It is easy to become preoccupied with the tasks of living. I have also tried to help myself. Initially it helped to write down my thoughts and feelings; then I revised my journal to create a book in the hope that it would help other people who had also suffered a sudden, unexpected loss. Several readers have sent letters acknowledging that the book has helped them, and I am always grateful to hear it.

My wife and I have also invented rituals to commemorate Jason's life and to affirm our ongoing love for him. Every Christmas my wife decorates a small tree and we put it by his grave. Christmas was Jason's favorite holiday and in this way we include him in our celebration. Other rituals are less formal. Jason loved to light candles, so my wife keeps a candle at the grave and whenever she goes to the cemetery she lights it. It is not a religious act but simply a gesture of love and remembrance. One of my rituals is to pick up any coin I see on the ground and keep it in my pocket until the next time I visit the cemetery. Jason was careless with money and was always losing change. He would typically have coins lying on the floor of his car or his room, so when I find coins it's as if Jason is still alive, still losing money, and it's my job to return it to him. There is a small pile of coins on the family monument next to Jason's name.

One problem with such rituals is that they are "public." Rituals done in the privacy of your home are safe, but creating a ritual in a public place like the cemetery makes you vulnerable and you must accept that. On one visit to Jason's grave I noticed that the two or three dollars worth of change that I had left there was gone. Instead of feeling angry, I was sorry that someone had been reduced to such a state that they had to steal a few coins left by a grave. But I continue to bring Jason "his" lost change. Far more difficult than someone taking the coins was the theft of the Christmas tree we always place by Jason's grave, primarily because several ornaments had much sentimental value. My wife wrote a letter to the local paper telling the thief to enjoy the tree for the holidays but to return the ornaments so we could use them again. There was no response.

Jan and I had discussed the possibility of vandalism or someone stealing ornaments, so we were prepared in case that happened. We did not think anyone would steal a decorated Christmas tree next to a grave, but we understood that placing the tree there made us susceptible to intentional misbehavior or thoughtless pranks. Although the theft of the tree upset us, the anticipation of problems helped us respond to the theft—placing another tree beside Jason's grave. Instead of decorations we attached notes to its branches asking the thief to return the ornaments, but they were never returned. One of Jason's former high school classmates had read Jan's letter in the local newspaper and sent us an ornament. It was a gracious and generous gesture. The next year his ornament was among the newly purchased ornaments decorating the tree.

The Christmas tree was the basis for another ritual for me. During that first Christmas after Jason's death, I went to the cemetery almost every day. On one visit I noticed ticket stubs from a local movie theater stuck onto some branches among the other ornaments. Jason and his friends loved films, so I was certain that some of them had stopped at the cemetery on their way back from a film and impulsively stuck the ticket stubs on the branches. I liked the idea and brought my own ticket stubs to attach to the tree. For the months when there is no tree there, I stuff the ticket stubs inside a small ceramic dog that guards Jason's grave.

My wife has developed private rituals as well. Each time she visits the cemetery she kisses her fingers and brushes them against the picture of Jason on the stone saying, "I love you, Jason. I miss you." She also keeps some of Jason's sweaters in a drawer, and when she is really missing him and wishing for a hug from him, she will wear one of his sweaters. One of the several items recovered from the car after the accident was an L.L. Bean backpack that Jason used for carrying his schoolbooks. It was returned to us at the hospital that night, and we take that backpack with us whenever we leave for a long trip. It is a way to pretend that he is with us.

Such rituals have helped me heal. I am better than I was.

Immediately after Jason's death there was a period of numbness. When the numbness receded and the pain increased, I sometimes used alcohol to bring the numbness back. After each day at work I would come home and write in my journal, desperately trying to capture my pain in words. Afterwards I would watch television or read, but too many times I would open a bottle of wine and drink until the numbness returned. It was a bad idea, but it took a while for me to recognize how harmful it was. Sometimes alcohol did not even offer an illusion of relief, and then I would listen to certain songs whose words would make me weep. Tears helped far more than alcohol, working like a safety valve, they provided a release from the painful pressure welling up in my heart.

I am better now than I was.

For a long time after Jason's death, it still felt like the accident had happened yesterday. Many months passed before it began to feel like the accident had happened last week. Years passed before it seemed like the accident had happened last month. It is now 8 years since Jason's death and it feels like the accident happened a few months ago. This slow passage of my internal clock suggests how raw the wound is and how much it still hurts, but it is also a measure of the healing that has occurred.

Much of the healing has come from the rituals we have invented: the candles and Christmas trees and coins. Much of it has come from my writing and the stories about Jason that I continue to tell. Much of it has come from the openness with which my wife and I talk about Jason or about those moments when our grief overwhelms us in a rush of memory and regrets and tears. Such moments are often predictable, but occasionally they catch us by surprise.

One time I was invited to speak to a Compassionate Friends group about my grief experience and my book. As the meeting began, everyone sat in a circle, and when the grieving parents introduced themselves they gave the name of the child they lost as well as the names of their other children. Thinking about what to say, I thought I was prepared when it was my turn. I talked about Jason's death when he was 19 years old, and I said I also had a daughter who had "just turned 20 which made her mother and I very happy." While saying those last few words, my throat tightened, my voice quavered and my eyes welled up with tears. Those words caused a wave of emotion to surge through me, and I suddenly realized just how important this particular birthday was.

The healing goes on, as do the rituals. And I am better now than I was.

Despite the improvement, there are still times when I am reminded of an experience from my adolescence that was described in my book *The Fall of a Sparrow* (1994). My father's job was to pick up dead animals from area farms and take them to a factory where they were skinned and the meat was processed into dog food. At one particular farm, my father had been told to pick up a calf that had just died:

> The cattle were clustered in groups. My father drove toward a cow standing alone near her calf and licking it. The mother was doing all that she could to comfort the calf, to heal it, to make it well, but the calf was dead. The calf looked pretty small, so my father asked me to help him pick it up. This would save some time. When we drove up next to the calf, the mother moved away, but not far away. She watched as my father let down the rear gate of the truck; she watched as my father and I grabbed her calf by the legs and threw it into the truck; she watched as my father and I closed and locked the rear gate.
>
> My father had to turn around and drive out the way we came, so I rolled down my window and watched the mother slowly walk back to where her calf had been. She sniffed the empty spot, then looked up at the departing truck. She began to run. At first I thought she was running after the truck, but she was running in a circle around the calfless spot. She ran in ever widening circles while we drove out of the pasture. (1994, pp. 135-136)

It is still a vivid scene in my memory, and I have always thought that the mother was doing a dance of grief. It feels like that when my mind is spinning in circles of thought about Jason, wondering where he would be living and what he would be doing if he had not died on September 13. Watching a movie, I wonder if he would have liked it, and I wonder if he would have realized his dream of making movies.

Such thoughts continue dancing round and round the empty space of his absence in ever widening circles.

I am better now than I was, but there is no antidote for grief.

The son I loved is dead. That fact is as cold and hard as the granite that marks his grave. My grief will be as permanent as that stone on which my name is carved next to his. I still grieve for Jason because I still miss him, and I will miss him until I am lying next to him. But Jason loved life, and he would not want me to waste what's left of mine. He would want me to be actively involved in my work and in activities with my family, appreciating the joy that life offers.

So I go on, embracing Jason's memory because he is my partner in this endless dance of grief. Although saddened by the absence of my son, I am grateful for the presence of my wife and daughter. My love for Jason can cause some suffering, but it is also part of the cure as I continue learning how to use this love in a positive way.

Because I know that is possible, I am better than I was.

REFERENCES

Cioran, Emile. Emile M. Cioran quotes. www.icelebz.com/quotes/emile-m-cioran

Eliot, T. S. (1967). Burnt Norton section of The Four Quartets. In S. Bradley, R. C. Beatty, & E. H. Long (Eds.), *The American tradition in literature.* New York: W. W. Norton & Company, Inc.

Koppelman, K. (1994). *The fall of a sparrow: Of death, dreams, and healing.* Amityville, NY: Baywood.

Thompson, Francis Daisy. (1919). *Complete poetical works of Francis Thompson* (p. 1). New York: Boni and Liveright, Inc.

CHAPTER 4

Reconciliation: Living with an Absence

One thing is certain and the rest is lies,
The flower that once has bloomed forever dies.
            Edward FitzGerald (1965, p. 60)

The most difficult part of bereavement for me has been accepting this void, this absence in my daily life. For a brief period I pretended there was an alternate universe somewhere and my son escaped into it. In this alternate universe, Jason was able to do all the things he should have done during his life in this universe—finishing college, falling in love, getting married, pursuing a career, having children, growing old, and enjoying grandchildren. In this alternate reality, I did not attend his funeral; instead, he attended mine. I liked this fantasy because my reality seemed surreal. My fantasy of an alternate universe made much more sense, even though it was just a fantasy.

> There are dreams stronger than death.
> Men and women die holding these dreams.
>   Carl Sandburg

In the normal logic of life, an absence should mean a lighter load, perhaps less responsibility. But when a loved one is absent, it creates a burden much harder to bear, and Jason's absence was such a burden. Fortunately, a person doesn't carry this weight around constantly. At work, there were constant demands related to teaching and other responsibilities or just talking with students or colleagues; and at home much time was taken up with reading or writing or even watching television. Most of the time I did not feel burdened by grief, but if something happened to remind me of Jason, the load was quickly shifted onto my shoulders once again. Being reminded of my son could involve something as simple as seeing a student who looked like Jason or hearing someone call out the name Jason; it might be a boy in a grocery store calling for his father or hearing a certain song on the radio. No matter where or when or how it happened, I had to adjust to the burden and refocus on what I was doing.

> It is as natural to die as to be born, and to a little infant, perhaps, the one is as painful as the other.
> Francis Bacon

In a few conversations following my son's death, people tried to console me with a popular sentiment that "God only gives burdens to people that they can bear." I did not find this consoling. What did they mean? How was I supposed to interpret the statement? Does it mean that God selected my son for an early death because God knew that I could "handle it?" Am I to assume that if I had been a weaker man, God would have selected someone else's son and let Jason live? If I believed that, it would add such guilt to the feelings of loss that my grief would be even harder to bear.

I wondered why people would say this, or why they would believe it was true. The only purpose for expressing such a belief would seem to be to console the person saying it—assuring them that their God was a just God, and that there had to be some purpose, some kind of sense, even in a seemingly senseless death. Because I did not have a conventional belief in God, this was not the kind of sentiment that would help me feel better about my son's death. Perhaps people wanted me to believe the cliché that "God is in His Heaven and all is right in the world," but all was not right in my world. There was no purpose that God or any human being could devise to justify my son's death.

> That man who is from God sent forth,
> Doth yet again to God return?—
> Such ebb and flow must ever be,
> Then wherefore should we mourn?
> William Wordsworth

People who have lost a loved one, especially a child, often share my frustration with such "sympathy." I have talked to various people about their grief experience, and I have learned valuable lessons from all of them, but after many conversations, I have realized that there is no magic trick, no secret strategy. When people have described their efforts to be reconciled to their loss, I have often wondered if their grief was similar to mine, and if what they did would help me. A poem by Emily Dickinson describes her encounters with grieving individuals and the tendency to compare our grief with others:

> I measure every grief I meet
>   With analytic eyes;
> I wonder if it weighs like mine
>   Or has an easier size. . . .
> I wonder if it hurts to live,
>   And if they have to try,
> And whether, could they choose between,
>   They would not rather die.

On a fundamental level, any parent struggling with the death of a child might wish that he or she were dead. Parents may say that they would have taken their child's place if they had been given a choice, but we don't have that choice. As I mourned the loss of my son, several people commended me for having the "courage" to go on. This seems like such a strange comment. In my experience, the people perceiving bereaved parents as courageous are usually people who have not suffered such a loss. They often say that they could not imagine what it would be like to lose a child and that they did not believe they could have coped with such a loss. I know they meant this as a compliment, but such comments only reveal a lack of understanding of the reality of loss. Bereaved parents have to go on, not out of courage but from necessity.

> Time does not heal, but it helps you to accept the pain that you're feeling.
>   Earl Grollman

Conte Vittorio Alfieri argued that in certain situations, "The test of courage is not to die but to live" (1979, p. 120). Perhaps perceiving bereaved parents as courageous expresses a similar sentiment, but dying would literally mean committing suicide. How can that be regarded as a realistic choice? Individuals suffering a loss still have other people in their lives. I had a wife and another child; I had parents and siblings. Every semester new students came to my classes, and throughout my teaching career I have experienced a sense of satisfaction and accomplishment. There were many reasons to go on living. Because of those reasons, it is not accurate to describe my actions in response to Jason's death as illustrating a display of courage. I simply did what had to be done, and that included accepting his death and finding a way to live in his absence.

There were many activities that helped me to accept my loss. Collecting, printing, and distributing Jason's writing to family members and friends; placing a Christmas tree by his grave each year; creating a scholarship fund in his memory; writing letters to several famous people he admired to thank them for being a positive force in Jason's life. Other grieving parents have engaged in activities for whatever measure of relief such activities could bring. There was one difference in my experience that occurred. Garrison Keillor responded to my letter with an offer to perform a benefit to raise money for Jason's scholarship fund. Thanks to that benefit, scholarships in Jason's name have been given every year since he died. My wife and I have personally attended the awards ceremony to hand out a simulated Oscar statue and the scholarship check to the recipients.

Such activities illustrate efforts to become reconciled to Jason's death. After my book was published, I shared my grief experience at bereavement conferences, including a few held outside the United States in Canada and Israel. Attending these conferences has been valuable because of the insights offered there, not only from people on their own grief journey, but professionals with knowledge of different aspects of bereavement and grief, such as ministers, rabbis, researchers, teachers, funeral home directors, and hospice workers. These people are among the most compassionate human beings I have ever had the privilege to know, and I always come away from these conference experiences feeling nurtured and affirmed.

> The great tragedy of life is not that some men perish, but that they cease to love.
> W. Somerset Maugham

The examples from wisdom literature on reconciliation begin with the boxed text containing Carl Sandburg's suggestion that love may transcend death as he encourages us to embrace our individual dreams or the dreams we share with those we love. Francis Bacon insists that death is as natural a part of life as being born, but he says nothing about an afterlife. By contrast, William Wordsworth argues that if a Creator sent us into the world, then surely we must return to that Creator when we depart from it. Although Earl Grollman refutes the cliché that "time heals all wounds," he also offers the assurance that the passage of time can lead to reconciliation. Somerset Maugham reminds us that the greatest reconciliation we can achieve is to love others for the entire time we have between birth and death.

One of the most important insights from attending bereavement conferences was the emphasis on remembering as a way to heal. This insight was the inspiration for the poem "In Your Absence." The poem begins by describing the pain that initially accompanies a loss, especially the sense of loneliness that loss brings. Even during shopping trips to the mall or at a party surrounded by people, a grieving person is aware of who is missing. This awareness can have a chilling effect that only becomes stronger in those moments when one is actually alone. Although the pain of a loss cannot be eradicated, it can be alleviated by the use of memory as expressed in the final verses of the poem.

The essay "For Those Who Stand and Wait" perhaps best expresses the sense of reconciliation I have managed to achieve since my son's death. The essay does not offer easy answers for dealing with grief, but it describes a point in my journey where I had begun to accept Jason's death. Part of that acceptance was influenced by what I learned from the stories and experiences of others. My grief journey began with my son's fatal car accident, and though it will continue until my death, the end of the essay describes a path that I continue to explore intellectually and spiritually. I'm not sure where the path will lead, but I am on it now and will follow where it takes me.

IN YOUR ABSENCE

Loneliness
Flopped on my lap
    like a snowball
    (so I picked it up
    and ran my hands over it).

It was very firm and very cold,
The kind cruel children make,
    packing and squeezing
    until the ball is hard enough
    to hurt when it hits.

With absent-minded curiosity
    I held it a long time—
Until I felt the coldness of it
    numbing my fingers,
    sending swift messengers
    whispering frantically,
      "Let it go."

And though I did,
    the numbness remained.
I walked into the kitchen
    to make some tea—
That should warm me up
    (I thought).

But neither the steam
    (from the kettle)
Nor the hot liquid
    (swallowed carefully)
Nor the warmed cup
    (Held with both hands)
Could thaw me,
    (although now my hands
    and lips were warm).

I put the cup down and
    walked to the couch.

Picking up some pillows
    I punched them,
    all of them,
        again and again
        but it did no good.

So I stopped struggling
    and lay down,
    letting the chilling numbness
    spread through me.

Shivering in silence
    I soon fell asleep,
    and was warmed
        by dreams
        of you.

FOR THOSE WHO STAND AND WAIT

> Let me tell you something . . . I'm not done
> grieving yet, and I don't care who knows it!

The tombstone makes no response. Of course, I wasn't really talking to it. I was simply talking out loud and it was simply there, mute as always. It was Sunday. It was a sunny Sunday and I had decided to drive around for a while. I like to do that on the weekend when it's sunny and warm. I drive around and notice what other people are doing. On this particular day I saw two children playing on the swings at one of the city's parks. Their mothers sat on a bench talking and laughing because it was Sunday and the sun was shining and their kids were playing and it's still too early for mosquitoes.

Before returning home, I like to stop at Oak Grove Cemetery to visit my "family." That's how I think of them, like an extended family. There's Baby Harley with the toy trucks he must have liked to play with nestled next to the stone with his name and dates. There's Katie with three balloons carved on her stone, floating above her forever, each one representing two years of her brief life. There are graves of Civil War soldiers here, and flags next to many more tombstones. I nod my head solemnly for the veterans of these wars, foreign and domestic. Many of the markers for Moms and Dads say "Parents of . . ." and list the names of their children. It is a statement about legacy as these stones quietly insist: whatever else we were, whatever else we did, the best thing about our lives was the children we leave behind.

Some markers whisper clues to passing strangers to provoke speculation about their story. A man born in 1949 died in 1982, and the name next to his was a boy born in 1975 who died in 1991—just 16, just beginning a life. Is this a father and son lying next to each other? Did the father die in an accident? Did the son share a similar fate or did he take his own life? Whatever the truth of this tale, it is a tragic one. Somewhere a wife and mother lives with a heavy heart. Were there brothers and sisters? The stone doesn't say.

One thing I do know about the people in this cemetery is that most of them were white, but such things as race or gender or social class don't matter much here. Death is the great equalizer and this is the promised paradise, a place of harmony where the Lyon lies down with the Lamb. A few huge monuments proclaim the names of Hixon or Hood, attempting to maintain the dignity and status that money provided during their lifetime, but big or small, the markers have the same message: beneath this stone is the remains of a life where no life remains.

Although there is racial homogeneity, there is some ethnic diversity. Anderson and Johnson and Peterson and Sorenson give proof of Swedish migration, and Lars Hagen's stone states quite unequivocally that he was born in "Norge" but died an American. I cannot guess the origin of Abplanalp until I read the text below one name on this family monument, "*Hier ruht unser lieber Bruder.*" Under the German name on one slate stone are the words "*Mein Herz,*" but there are no names or dates there. Was this an individual, a family? The grave does not yield its secrets but preserves the mystery of its occupants (or occupant).

There are more German names: Rademacher and Strauss and Molzohn . . . and Koppelman. And there is my son among this family of strangers. Jason David Koppelman—born 1970, died 1989. Whenever I feel moved to protest this outrageously short time, other graves remind me that many have had even fewer years. A small stone announces that Mary Ellen was born and died on the same day: January 2, 1933. The same parents gave birth to Elizabeth Ann who lived just three days. There are no graves in the large gap between these small stones. I like to think those plots were for the children who survived, and who survive still.

I am reminded of my own status as a survivor every time I come here. Next to Jason's name is my wife's name and then my name, with birth dates recorded and death dates yet unknown. It is strange to see your name on such a stone, a preview of coming attractions. This is where my body will be someday. Is there something more to me, something like a spirit or a soul that will transcend the death of my body? I can't be certain, and I certainly can't know what it is or what it does. I doubt that I will ever "know" because even if something survives the death of the body, there is no guarantee that individual consciousness survives with it.

It is a mystery. We all speculate and debate, but I do not have enough confidence to be sure of any answer. I keep asking questions. Although we are provided with clues, it is probably a mystery that will never be solved. One such clue from my experience is a story I have told before, but a few more details have been added here for purposes of clarity. This is my contribution to the debate and to the mystery.

At Jason's funeral, my wife and daughter sat on either side of me in the family section, an empty chair next to my daughter as if we expected our son to join us. The coffin was the center of attention for the mourners, the family merely a sideshow of grief. We sat there wishing we didn't have to be here, wishing there was no need to have a funeral. My wife was dreading the moment when we would stand by the empty grave at the cemetery with Jason's coffin poised over it, ready to be lowered after everyone left. When the music began, an anonymous organist on tape playing "In the Garden," it was neither inspirational nor comforting. Twitching in the chair, I was feeling guilty about selecting this music. I should have listened to the recorded selections before the funeral to be sure of its quality. Jason would have hated such passionless music.

Suddenly the door leading out to the parking lot slammed open as if a child had impetuously dashed out of the room. My wife and daughter had the same thought I did, something that was Jason—call it soul or spirit—had just left. Our sense that he was no longer present seemed to allow us to breathe again and to grieve, knowing that the grief would now help us deal with his absence, today and in the days to come. There have been other moments when I have had a sense of Jason's presence for a few fleeting seconds, but the closed door bursting open on a calm, autumn day was the only time there was tangible evidence of something. Although the memory remains vivid, I am still not certain what to make of it. Even though it does not prove the existence of an immortal soul, it gave comfort to those who witnessed it, and the memory comforts us still.

Since then I have had to adjust to my fate, going on with this ongoing grief. I often think of the expression, "a fate worse than death." What does that mean? When you die, your suffering is done, so any "fate" that keeps you alive makes you vulnerable to pain, loss, heartache. If you lose a child or anyone you love, you are guaranteed to suffer. It is measured out daily by the teaspoon or tablespoon. Is this a fate worse than death?

I am thinking of this while standing before my son's grave, quiet now, tired of talking. An older man is riding an old bicycle on one of the paved paths winding through the cemetery. He is large; he dwarfs the bicycle. He has a sleeping bag, rolled up and tightly tied, hanging from the right handlebar, and a dirty blue duffle bag whose handle he holds in his left hand. He ignores me, but he looks around intently as if he is lost or is looking for something—a place to sleep perhaps. I watch him bike slowly, looking thoughtfully at the tombstones. He will be back. I am sure of it. After all, a cemetery is a place of rest. He will be safer here than at one of the parks; the police will not come here to roust him out. He can rest with the other sleepers, quiet companions who will not bother him. Perhaps he also thinks of them as family.

I wondered if he knew about the animals. The cemetery is next to a wetlands area; I have seen beavers and deer and other creatures in the cemetery. Driving through at dusk I have seen animals hiding among the stones, darting across the road, betrayed briefly in my headlights as they seek the safety of the swamp. In the winter I have seen their tracks in the snow near Jason's grave. I don't think they will bother the stranger. They will probably stay away from his sleeping spot wherever he decides that will be. It is his fate, apparently, to be homeless. Is his a fate worse than death? It would seem not. He continues to live, even if it means sleeping in a graveyard. And so do I, even if it means coming to a graveyard to be "with" the son I cannot be with. Survivors do what we have to do, trying to find reasons to go on.

In his novel *Mother Night*, Kurt Vonnegut (1999) invents a double agent who pretends to be a Nazi during World War II so he can spy for the allies, cleverly sending information encoded in the Nazi propaganda he writes. After the war, the CIA tells him they do not want to inform the public about the true nature of his role during the war for fear he will be a target for assassination by those he betrayed. While trying to create a new life for himself, he stumbles into a meeting of militant Zionists who recognize him and attack him. He is rescued by neo-Nazis who have been monitoring the Zionist meeting and intervene to help him escape. They take him out a side door to the sidewalk, then they reenter the building to rejoin their colleagues who are assaulting the Zionists. At that moment this man's life seems so strange, so surreal, so pointless, that he cannot think of a reason to leave. He can think of no place to go, nor any purpose for going, so he simply stands there on the sidewalk. A police officer comes along and asks what he is doing there. He says nothing, just stands there and shakes his head. The officer says, "Move along," and so he does.

Anyone who has struggled with the loss of a loved one knows this feeling. There are days when you simply go on doing what you do out of a sense of habit, just following the routine, just putting one foot in front of the other. Ultimately you must find better reasons to go on, but it is not easy. For a long time I kept wishing that Jason was still alive, wishing and wanting it with such a ferocious desire that I did not know what to do about the frustration and pain it caused me. Listening to music or the passive activity of watching television would sometimes distract me. And sometimes I sought solace in the solitude of drink. It would dull my senses enough to give me peace, even if it was only the illusion of peace, even if only for a few hours before succumbing to sleep. In the morning I would get up and begin another day. I put one foot in front of the other in response to a voice in my own head that said, "Move along."

In the midst of this struggle I remembered something I had read years ago in a book on world religions. The chapter on Buddhism had discussed how to deal with desire. I found the book and reread the chapter. It said that desire actually consisted of two components: the desire for the thing itself, and the desire that this desire be fulfilled. Buddhists believe that people cannot stop desiring things, it is part of our nature, but it is possible to control the desire that one's desire be fulfilled. That made sense. I stopped trying to control my desperate longing for Jason to be alive so I could hug him and tell him how much I loved him. I indulged in that desire whenever I felt like it, understanding that this desire was a reflection of my love for my son. At the same time I kept reminding myself that what I wanted was not going to happen. This seemed to help me. I wanted to feel that emotion because it allowed me to express my love for Jason. I didn't want to bottle my love up and hide it away, but I didn't want to be irrational about my desire being satisfied. This insight also helped me to write about my grief, putting words on paper to capture the pain and also to express my love for my son.

After writing for several months about my grief experiences, I sent some excerpts to a friend who was a minister in San Antonio. I was coming to San Antonio in a few weeks to attend a conference, and he invited me to stay with him. He also invited me to meet with some members of his church who had formed a "grief group." He thought it would be helpful if I shared with them the grief experiences described in my writing. In my preparations for the meeting, I decided to begin with the dream that I had a week after Jason died, since that dream was the beginning of my healing process.

We met on a Saturday morning: two men and about a dozen women, most of them Mexican American. I began by describing the first few days after Jason's accident when I experienced numbness, a sense of being burdened by a heavy weight, and not getting enough sleep because I kept waking up early. Admitting my doubts about the existence of God, I told them of my desperate prayer for help, how I fell asleep and dreamed about Jason. I described the surprising energy I felt throughout the following day and how I began sleeping normally. They listened intently, nodding their heads sympathetically until the description of the conversation with my doctor who suggested I had experienced a clinical depression that may have been diminished by certain chemicals stimulated by my dream. At that point some of the Mexican American women looked down at the floor and others smiled at me the way a knowing mother smiles at her child. Afterwards my friend thanked me for coming and said the group benefited from my visit, "except for the part where the doctor explained your dream." He knew they could not accept the doctor's explanation because they had their own, an explanation he had learned from working with Native American and Mexican American communities for the past 14 years. They believed in spirits that survived the body's death, and that these spirits could come to someone in a dream. "You needed to see Jason, so his spirit came to you in your dream. His spirit healed you and allowed you to get on with your life."

I wanted to believe what these women believed. It is a more comforting belief than the doctor's explanation, but I'm a product of my culture. It's not easy to abandon an insistence on scientific explanations. I don't read horoscopes; I would not phone a psychic. I demand proof, evidence, a rational basis for belief. Yet I know that life is not always rational. There are mysteries that cannot be solved, questions that can never be answered. We have a consciousness we carry with us throughout our lives. Where was this consciousness before we were born? Where is it after we die? These are matters of faith. We choose to believe in certain answers and live our lives as if they were true. I want to have a faith that says I will see my son again. Can I have such a faith? Can I believe in spirits like the Mexican American women? Can I embrace this truth as confidently as they do? Perhaps, but I cannot do this right now, not yet.

I told a friend who works with me at the university about the grief group in San Antonio. Dan is a Native American and he shared the perspective of the women in the grief group. He said a belief in spirits is common among Native Americans, and the idea that the spirit of a loved one could visit someone in a dream was more than just a matter of belief for him. He told me this story.

Before Dan had even dated the woman he eventually married, she had a dream where a stout, older Indian woman came to her with a basket, saying sternly, "You have work to do," admonishing her to get to it. Laura had no idea what to make of this dream. When she began dating Dan, he told her about Beverly, his mother, and what an important person she had been in his life. Laura had noticed a number of framed photographs of Beverly in Dan's apartment. After they got married, Laura started to tell Dan about her strange dream where an older woman came to her, but Dan interrupted, "It was my mother." The thought came to him the moment she began talking about this dream.

Laura argued that it couldn't have been his mother because the woman in the dream was very stout and in his pictures Beverly was thin and beautiful. Dan said those pictures were taken when she was younger, but his mother had gained a lot of weight before she died. Dan searched for a picture of his mother toward the end of her life, and when he showed one to Laura, she said immediately, "That's the woman." Dan believed that the basket in her dream referred to the grandchild his mother wanted, so when they had their first child, a baby girl, they named her Beverly. Although Laura's dream suggests that a soul or spirit may survive death, there are other explanations. I can draw no conclusions, but such experiences reinforce a sense of wonder, a sense of possibility in the mystery that surrounds life and death.

Late one night I received a phone call from my cousin, a Presbyterian minister, who had also lost his son several years ago. He called to tell me of the unusual experience that occurred during his recent back surgery. Before the operation he was given an anesthetic, and as the drug took effect he began to see shapes that became gradually more distinct. He didn't know if he was dreaming or having a vision, but he saw our grandmother who had died almost 30 years ago. On one side of her was his son, and on the other side was my son. There were many details in this dream and he remembered them clearly in his description. Toward the end of the dream, Jason said to him, "tell my Dad not to worry about me," and that I should "look at page 875 in the Bible." When my cousin finished his description of the dream, he said that was all he wanted to say for now. Before he hung up I wanted to make sure I had the right page number, so I deliberately gave him the wrong number, asking if it was page 835. He corrected me—page 875.

I thought about this curious reference. It is far more common to cite a book of the Bible by the chapter and verse, like John 3:16. Of course, Jason wouldn't know that because he did not go to Sunday school or church. I have five Bibles, each of which is a different translation, so I wondered which Bible I should use. It occurred to me that the page number might refer to the passage from Matthew where God is described as concerned even for the fall of a sparrow; that passage was the basis for the title of my book about Jason's death. I grabbed my King James Bible and found the passage in Matthew, but it was on page 10 because the pagination started over where the New Testament began. I wondered if the last page of the Old Testament was 865 since that would make the tenth page of Matthew the 875th page, but the last page of the Old Testament in that Bible was 848. There was no page 875.

I wanted to make sense of this. Why was I given a page number? With a chapter and verse reference I could look up the passage in any Bible. Being given a page number suggested that I would need to look in a particular Bible. Which of the several translations should I use? I wasn't sure. Why did this have to be so confusing? Why didn't Jason just show up in one of my dreams and tell me what he wanted me to hear? Why was he in my cousin's dream? I was even starting to feel a little resentful that Jason did not come to me in this dream but appeared in my cousin's dream, and that was when I remembered my cousin's gift.

When Jason graduated from high school, my cousin sent him a gift that ministers often send on such occasions—a Bible. I knew immediately that this was the Bible that must be used to locate page 875. I found the Bible on a shelf in Jason's old room under several other books. It was the "New International Version," which included extensive footnotes, so after 800 pages, this Bible was only up to the Psalms. On page 875, two-thirds of the page was devoted to footnotes, but on that page Psalm 84 began:

> How lovely is your dwelling place
> O Lord Almighty!
> My soul yearns, even faints,
> for the courts of the Lord;
> my heart and my flesh cry out
> for the living God.
> Even the sparrow has found a home,
> and the swallow a nest for herself . . .

Had my sparrow found a home, a haven? Was Jason trying to tell me this, using an indirect means to deliver this message in order to be all the more convincing? There are no definitive answers to these questions. They must be answered by faith. If I believe my son was trying to reassure me, then that becomes my truth. I can believe in a God who creates an immortal soul in each of us that will return to its creator after the body dies. I can choose to believe, knowing that my belief may not be true.

This is my challenge: to be a person of faith I must choose to believe in the context of doubt, to embrace a possibility as if it were a truth. It is not easy. I have not mastered this challenge yet, and perhaps I never will. Instead, the person from the gospels who seems most like a kindred spirit is the father in the fourth chapter of Mark who brings his sick child to Jesus to be healed. Unlike that father, I do not come with a living child in my arms. I come with the lifeless body of a child flung into a ditch whose shattered skull leaked his life into the ground on the darkest night of my life. And when Jesus says to that father, and to all of us, "All things are possible to him who believes," I feel my heart sink as I wrestle with my fears and doubts, as did the father who stood before Jesus. But I take some comfort in that father's response, and echo his reply:

> Lord I believe, help thou my unbelief.

So here I stand at this point in my grief journey, with thousands of faithful fathers and mothers who have lost a child and struggle with despair. The questions are hard. The answers are not easily found. I search for a faith that will be nurturing and comforting. I want to believe that my son knows of my love for him, and that at some time, in some place, he will come to me, knowing how much that will comfort me. I can only believe, placing a welcome mat before the doorway to dreams, keeping the fire of love going in my heart, hoping for that special guest to surprise me with his presence. Waiting.

NOTES

1. The title of this essay refers to John Milton's Sonnet XIX ("When I Consider...") that concludes with the following lines:

> **God doth not need**
> Either man's work or his own gifts; who best
> Bear his mild yoke, they serve him best; his State
> Is Kingly. Thousands at his bidding speed
> And post o'er Land and Ocean without rest:
> They also serve who only stand and wait.

2. The chapter on Buddhism was in *The Religions of Man* by Huston Smith, a wonderful book first published by Harper & Row in 1958.

REFERENCES

Alfieri, Conte Vittorio. (1979). *Peter's quotations: Ideas for our times* (p. 120). L. Peter (Ed.). New York: Bantam Books.
Dickinson, Emily. (1959). I measure every grief I meet. In R. N. Linscott (Ed.), *Selected poems and letters of Emily Dickinson* (p. 136). Garden City, NY: Doubleday/Anchor.
Fitzgerald, Edward. (1965). *The Rubaiyat of Omar Khayam* (p. 60). New York: Avon Books.
Koppelman, K. (1994). *The fall of a sparrow: Of death, dreams, and healing*. Amityville, NY: Baywood.
Smith, Huston. (1958). *The religions of man*. New York: Harper & Row.
Vonnegut, Jr., Kurt. (1999). *Mother night*. New York: Avon Books.

PART 3

Responding to Expected Deaths

I have heard it related of a poor harvester
who died in a hospital bed,
that when the priest went to anoint his hands
with the oil of extreme unction,
he refused to open his right hand
which clutched a few dirty coins,
not considering that very soon neither his hand
nor he himself would be his own any more.
And so we close and clench,
not our hand, but our heart,
seeking to clutch the world in it.

                    Miguel de Unamuno (1954, p. 42)
                          The Tragic Sense of Life

CHAPTER 5

Bereavement: Expecting Death

> *Death stands above me, whispering low*
> *I know not what into my ear;*
> *Of his strange language all I know*
> *Is, there is not a word of fear.*
> Walter Savage Landor (1965, p. 302)

Once as a young man, I remember riding in a car with my father when we somehow began to talk about death. After talking for a few minutes, we came to an intersection where we had to stop. Possibly sensing my feelings of uncertainty and anxiety, my father turned to look directly at me and said, "I'm not afraid to die." There was sincerity and conviction in his voice, and I admired him for being able to feel that way and to express it so resolutely.

I wanted to feel the same way—to accept the inevitability of death and not to fear it. Having become disenchanted with religion as an adult, I have tended to look for natural rather than supernatural explanations. I would like to be as rigorously logical as Arthur Schopenhauer, who said, "After your death you will be what you were before your birth," but I cannot yet accept this idea. It is not simply a fear of death that prevents me, but my personal sense of truth. I have always trusted my intuitive reactions to statements or arguments from others. Schopenhauer's statement seems possible, even probable, but my intuitive sense of truth has never affirmed it. What I am left with instead is a question: What are human beings supposed to do with the knowledge that we are going to die? I have continued to read philosophers, poets, theologians, and even scientists to discover what they have to say about death and what they think will happen after we die.

> Man is the only animal that contemplates death, and also the only animal that shows any sign of doubt of its finality.
> William Ernest Hocking

I have appreciated the insights of poets most of all. Many lines of poetry from Robert Frost, Emily Dickinson, and Walt Whitman (to name a few) have seemed "truth-full" and satisfying. Sometimes I just appreciate a metaphor, as when e. e. cummings (1954) describes death as life's "rhythmic lover," or when he suggests that: "life's not a paragraph/And death I think is no parenthesis." I have also read descriptions of how other cultures view death, and I have appreciated these diverse perspectives, especially those expressed in many Native American cultures. The following example is attributed to a Mohican chief called Aupumut, but it is one of many statements describing a similar attitude toward death expressed by many other American Indian cultures:

> When it comes time to die, be not like those whose hearts are filled with the fear of death, so when their time comes they weep and pray for a little more time to live their lives over again in a different way. Sing your death song, and die like a hero going home.

Unfortunately, I am not yet the hero Chief Aupumut challenges me to be. I have not only felt afraid about my own death, I have been worried for my family and friends. The poem "Night Visitor" is included in this chapter, because it illustrates that fear of death, describing death as a mysterious being lurking in the shadows, a presence from childhood reflecting a Halloween image. In contrast to this nightmarish vision, in my dreams death always occurs as an event rather than being personified as it was for me as a child. As a child, death was usually some kind of monster pursuing me, but as an adult, dreams of dying typically place me in a dangerous situation from which there is no apparent escape. And yet, in some of these dreams I manage to escape, usually by flying. Perhaps the ability to fly in these dreams can be interpreted as a subconscious belief in the possibility of surviving death, in the existence of an afterlife.

> Be of good hope in the face of death. Believe in this one truth for certain, that no evil can befall a good man either in life or death, and that his fate is not a matter of indifference to the gods.
>
> Socrates

For example, I have had numerous dreams where I am in a car, usually driving, and traveling down a treacherous, winding mountain road; for a variety of reasons—loss of brakes, icy road conditions—I cannot control the car as it hurtles off the road plummeting down a precipice. Prior to the car crashing and my apparently certain death, I often wake up, but sometimes I don't wake up. Sometimes when the car leaves the road it begins to fly, or I am thrown from the car and discover that I can fly. In either case, I survive.

Probably the strangest of such dreams was one where I had been thrown from the car and was gliding through the air rather than flying. In order for my body remain airborne, I had to hold both arms extended away from my body. While gliding slowly down toward earth, I noticed that the air was ruffling the sleeves of my long-sleeved shirt. I awoke to find myself sitting in bed and felt relieved. I noticed that my arms were still extended just as they had been in the dream, and then I saw that the sleeves of my pajamas were being ruffled just as the sleeves on my shirt had been ruffled in the dream where I was gliding. And then I actually did wake up, lying in bed on my side as usual. I have no explanation for the gliding dream, or for the dream within the dream.

The poetry concluding this chapter was written after the expected deaths of my sister, father, and mother. My sister Gay was 56 years old when she was diagnosed less than a month after Christmas with advanced colon cancer. The doctors said her cancer was so widespread they were not sure that she would make it to the next Christmas. Gay endured chemotherapy and radiation treatments, and through sheer determination she celebrated another Christmas with her grandchildren, and they celebrated several birthdays together (including one of her own) until she died shortly before her 58th birthday.

Because Gay was closer to my age than my other two sisters, we had a more intimate relationship as we were growing up, but as adults we grew further apart. To some degree this was due to the physical distance between us, and to some degree it was the difference in our personalities. Regardless of the reasons, as soon as I heard that Gay had cancer, my wife and I flew to California as soon as we could. After that first visit we went back as often as our work schedules and budget would allow. Gay didn't ask me to come, but it was the only thing I could do for her. When I was with her we did not speak of love or break into tears, because that was not how Gay and I had interacted in the past, and I was certain that she would be uncomfortable if I started doing that now. She understood that by coming to see her I was demonstrating my love for her, a love also expressed in the poem "Big Sisters," written shortly after she died.

The love we feel for others is what makes us most vulnerable and most human. I have always appreciated Christopher Morley's comment that "If we suddenly discovered that we had only five minutes left to say all we wanted to say, every telephone booth would be occupied by people trying to call up other people to stammer that they loved them." In this age of cell phones, the reference to a telephone booth may seem quaint, but no matter how the technology changes, the sentiment is still true.

> One dies only once, and it
> is for such a long time!
> Moliere

By the time Gay died, I could accept her death because she was in a lot of pain and was unable to do much for herself anymore. She did not even want her family to visit her. Hospice workers came to her home, and she appreciated the compassionate care they provided. They eased her pain and eased her way out of the world as well as they could. Gay had been active all her life, so being unable to get out of bed must have added insult to the injury of illness. As her life was ending, she was prepared to die. The same thing happened to my father-in-law. He was so miserable for the last few months of his life that he prayed every night for death to come in his sleep, and was disappointed each morning when he awoke. More compelling than any wisdom literature, these two experiences have demonstrated to me how someone could not only overcome the fear of death, but even welcome it, knowing that it would bring an end to suffering.

Although my father died a few months before my sister, his real death had occurred a few years earlier. Because of kidney failure, my father needed dialysis 3 days a week for the last 7 years of his life. This forced my parents to sell their house and leave the small town where they had always lived and where they raised their children. Roy and Lois moved to Iowa City, renting an apartment near the hospital that was also only about three blocks from the home of my oldest sister, Sally.

For reasons that still are unclear, Roy began to experience a slow but steady cognitive deterioration during the time he was on dialysis, and he became less physically energetic. He always read newspapers and kept up with the issues of the day, and he always had interesting insights to offer. Often he would see a humorous side to serious events that made me laugh, and all of this occurred in the context of his contagious *joie de vivre*. It was painful to watch that joy slowly dissipate. With each visit he talked less; more and more often I watched as my father slept in his chair. Even when he was awake he didn't have much to say, even when I peppered him with questions, so we watched a lot of television. Before long that sense of joy about life was gone. He merely persevered.

At this point my sister Sally sent a letter to all of her siblings describing a funeral she had recently attended. At the funeral, the children of the deceased father read letters thanking him for the many things he had done for them in their lives, as children and as adults. Sally was moved by their words, but she also thought it would have been better if the father could have read or heard these letters. Sally asked if we would be willing to write similar letters to our parents, describing what they had done for each of us and expressing our appreciation. Everyone thought it was a wonderful idea and we all agreed to send her our letters. Sally also requested that we send her old photographs so that she could create an album with our letters and photographs. She planned to present the album to our parents during a party to celebrate their birthdays—celebrated together since they were only a month apart.

After writing a rough draft of my letter, I read it aloud to my wife, asking her to suggest improvements. While reading about the role my father had played in my life and my profound sense of gratitude for all that he had done for me, tears ran down my face, and it took some time before I could stop weeping. I had been excited about the prospect of writing this letter, so the strong emotion that provoked these tears caught me off guard. After regaining some composure, I tried to understand what had just happened.

For the first time, I recognized that I had been feeling a form of grief for a long time without acknowledging it. This grief was a response to the loss of that personality who happened to be my father. As a boy and as a man I had always admired my father, as did many others. Roy's honesty and integrity were widely known and respected in his community. He was active in the local government and in his church. His gregarious personality attracted people. He was intelligent but not arrogant, and although he loved to talk, he was also a good listener. He was comfortable enough with his masculinity to express his emotions and could be moved to tears while watching a movie. He liked people and they liked him.

Much of my life had been a conscious effort to be the kind of man my father was. I was not as good at it as he was, but my life has been satisfying and certainly joy-full. Without realizing it, I had already been grieving what I had perceived as the gradual disappearance of this dynamic, thoughtful, exuberant man, but what I had written in my letter forcefully reminded me of his absence from my life. It was that sense of loss that had provoked the tears.

> Let us endeavor so to live, that when we die
> even the undertaker will be sorry.
> Mark Twain

For years after first encountering the poetry of Dylan Thomas, one of my favorite poems has been "Do Not Go Gentle Into That Good Night" (1957, p. 128). The lines of this poem that especially move me are from the refrain where he begs his father to resist death and insists that the old man standing on the precipice of death should "rage against the dying of the light." I felt this way about my father and hoped he would live for as long as possible, but the man that I had admired and respected was gone. Even though I could still see an image of him and I could put my arms around his body and express my love for him, the substance of the man no longer inhabited his body. His body was animated by breathing but not by Roy's unique spirit.

Being aware of these feelings, I assumed it would be easier to accept my father's death when it came, but it was not. I had just gone overseas to teach in a study-abroad program in Scotland when the phone call came from my sister saying that my father had died. I was calm at first because I knew this call would come one day, but now that it had come, my sense of loss intensified throughout the day. I was grieving Roy's death all over again. I grieved for the loss of the man and the loss of the father who had struggled to survive over the past several years, clinging to life largely for my mother's sake. He had always felt a responsibility to take care of her, even when she was taking care of him. Now he was gone. That day I began writing the poem that became "The Holy Grail" and would continue working on it for several weeks.

My wife and I flew back to Iowa to attend Roy's funeral. It was good to be with the gathering of family and friends who came to view the body and mourn the passing of this man. At the birthday party almost a year earlier Sally had presented my mother and father with the album of letters and pictures. Although Gay had not been able to come, the rest of the siblings came. Each of us read aloud our letter to our parents and Sally also read Gay's letter. My parents deeply appreciated the album but especially our letters; I was grateful to Sally for asking us to write them. That birthday party was one of the best celebrations that my parents would have during the last few years of their lives.

My father and sister died within five months of each other, and for a time the sense of loss seemed just as painful as the death of my son, but the pain was not as deep. It felt more like a bad bruise compared with the amputation that was my son's death. It did not take as long to recover from their loss because everyone knew these deaths were coming, just not the specific day and time. There was also a feeling that both of them had a "good death." For my sister, death brought an end to the pain and frustration of a bedridden existence during those final weeks. My father's death was peaceful, coming in the middle of the night with no sign of struggle. There had been opportunities for family members to be with my father and my sister, to show our love for them and to say goodbye before they left us to encounter whatever it is that happens once a life ends.

Similar feelings of loss came almost 2 years later when my mother died. Although they had loved each other for over 50 years, my father's death brought my mother a measure of relief, because Lois had largely borne the burden of caring for him in those final years when he was not able to be much of a companion. Many spouses who have had to be caretakers during the last years of their partner's life have felt a sense of relief when the spouse died. Some have felt guilty about having such feelings, but my mother did not feel guilty because she believed she had done as much as she could for Roy. She did not mind living alone, because she had never been a gregarious person. Sally would come over regularly and often helped Lois with her finances and shopping. Since it took only a few hours for me to drive to Iowa City, on several weekends my wife and I came down to visit her. My mother seemed content with this much companionship.

Lois had hoped to live a long and healthy life, but it was not to be. Shortly before my father died she was diagnosed with a form of leukemia that doctors said would become increasingly uncomfortable over time. They encouraged her to travel and play golf and engage in other physical activities while she still felt healthy. A few months after Roy's death, Lois boarded an airplane for the first time in her life and flew to Colorado to visit her sister. She took other trips, but before long she could not leave her apartment. The disease affected her organs, stretching her abdomen so much that it appeared to conceal a developing child instead of revealing the progress of her disease.

My sister kept me informed of my mother's condition, and her increasing discomfort. The greatest humiliation was when she needed help with some of her basic functions. Lois was 4 years younger than Roy, and she was angry at the thought that she was probably not going to live as long as he did, but as her suffering increased she became reconciled to her death. My wife and I were there the weekend that my mother died. The poems about my father and sister's death were written shortly after they died, but it took over a year before I could write about my mother's death. Perhaps "The Visit" took longer because my mother died the old-fashioned way—at home, surrounded by family. We're not used to that today. Perhaps more time was necessary to sort out the complex feelings that came from witnessing her final hours, something I had never done.

> Life is real! Life is earnest!
> And the grave is not its goal,
> Dust thou art to dust returneth,
> Was not spoken of the soul.
> Henry Wadsworth Longfellow

There is an extensive amount of wisdom literature addressing the expectation of one's own death and that of all human beings. Some of it involves advice on how to cope with this reality, but in the first boxed text provided in this essay, William Hocking chides those of us who still harbor illusions of an afterlife, while Socrates offers a rather vague assurance that a good life is not lived in vain. Moliere reminds us of the urgency of taking life seriously because of its brevity, while death, on the other hand, lasts eternally. Mark Twain uses humor to reinforce the words of Socrates, suggesting that we should try to live such a good life that even strangers will mourn our passing, but Henry Wadsworth Longfellow offers a passionate rejection of all doubts or fears of death with an exuberant and optimistic insistence on the existence of immortal souls destined for an afterlife that lies beyond the grave.

A final note about the poems: when writing poetry, I usually prefer to use standard poetic forms and rhymes, because I feel more confident working within a structure, but at times the emotion is too strong to be confined and words must be written without paying attention to structure. The poems that conclude this chapter may not necessarily represent good poetry in a literary sense, but they are an honest expression of grief over the loss of a loved one. The final poem in this chapter is my favorite of all four poems included here. I wish I could claim it as mine, but my sister Sally wrote "Swing Time," and for many reasons it seemed the best way to conclude this chapter.

NIGHT VISITOR

On this meandering journey of life,
   when disturbed by thoughts of death
I have read philosophy and poetry
   urging me to contemplate death as:
      a seductive temptress
      a soothing mother
      a satisfying lover.
But tonight . . . in bed . . . not sleeping,
   in a room three floors above ground,
I seemed to see a shapeless shadow
   just beyond my window.

It transformed into a human face,
   hideous, with empty eyes
   shallow as a pauper's grave.
A motionless face until a sudden smile
   revealed missing and broken teeth.
The head wagged back and forth,
   and I smelled the sickening scent
      of pity.

Half mad from fear, I leaped to my feet,
   cursing the face in the window . . .
When I approached the glass
   no image was reflected there,
Only a frosty fog remained
   from warm breath on the pane,
And I was not quite sure
      it was my own.

BIG SISTERS

One sister held and cuddled me,
  The other pushed and poked me.
One was passionate and tearful,
  The other was calm and resolute.
One sister showed me how to laugh,
  The other taught me to protect myself.

One sister offered the bittersweet juice of jazz;
  The other served up the spicy sauce of folk.
    (Miles Davis may have been cool,
      but Bob Dylan was hot . . .)
One sister applauded my deeds from the sidelines,
  The other challenged me in diverse arenas—
    a basketball court or a "friendly" retort.
      (I won some; I lost some . . .
      she was good.)

One sister lived near; we stayed connected.
  The other moved away; we stayed "in touch."
One sister was there for family events,
  The other received random photographs.
One sister warmly welcomed my frequent visits;
  The other hosted some sporadic appearances.

But the world descended down a dismal path;
  The distant sister—fatal victim of a sneak attack
    by the killer called colon cancer.

And so,
  sporadic visits speeded up
  clearly conscious of
    the revolution of earth
    and evolution of time
    and the devolution of her body
      shaking her spirit
      pulling her down
      taking her away
      too soon
      and forever
      and now . . .

My sister left her home today;
The sister everyone called Gay
  will now be gay no more.

I wrote some lines before she died,
No words of comfort came; I tried
   to say my heart was sore.

At times words simply can't reveal
   The way you feel;
They seem to mock us and conceal
   or sound bizarre.

Though products of nocturnal flights,
   we break away like satellites;
Yet we reflect their fading lights
   like distant stars.

Parental gifts passed on to me,
   transformed by sisters (partially)
     who taught me (inadvertently):

   to laugh and curse
     (in prose or verse)
   to be glad or perverse
   to scold or converse
   to expound or be terse
   to move on or reverse,

And my task has been
   to know just when
   to do each of them
     Based on the context
       or the pretext
       or the subtext.

But sister Gay's not here today.
It slipped away, the chance to say,
   "I love you (in my way)."

When last we hugged, I whispered,
   "Goodbye, take care."
   (Because I did love you . . .

   Even if I didn't say it,
And I think you knew that . . .
   Didn't you?)

THE HOLY GRAIL

"There's a message from your sister—"
"I'm so sorry that I missed her—"
"I'm so sorry that the message said
    your father's dead."

Bright bolts of lightning blast my brain
    while tardy thunder rumbles in my heart
    as day grows dark.

Water pools at the wells of my eyes—
    and when eyelids blink,
    as if a flag had fluttered,

Tears race down my cheeks
    to disappear within my beard
    where they wander, lost,
    never to emerge.
Did the sun drop?
Or did it stop . . .
    keeping a momentous silence
    before sinking soundlessly to sleep.

Whispering words I cannot hear,
    shadows surrender to the gloom
    of a darkness that had frightened me
    as a child.

But such shadows
    now beckon playfully,
Giving glimpses
    of a face—
    here and there—
    hiding behind veils;
      not monstrous
      or frightening.

More faces form—friendly, familiar,
    grandmothers and grandfathers
    uncles and aunts"
a nephew, a niece
a son . . .
and now a father.

All passed on—gone—resting.
I mimic them by pretending to sleep
    throughout a night in flight,
    but no peaceful rest is in it.

Alert at dawn,
Arriving to mourn
   a new death,
The old deaths still mourned
   even now.

The corpse looked cramped within the coffin—
Shoulders too big for such a box.
This wrinkled, ragged, worn-out body
   does not sleep either;
A sleeper moves and mumbles,
His breath brushes your face
   when you hover above his.
This body has passed the expiration date,
   Strange looking,
   Strange smelling,
As unfamiliar to the touch as a body bag
   stuffed with sand.

No blushes redden these cheeks,
No hearty handshakes left in these
   firm but frozen fingers.

I feel compelled to speak,
   to say "I love you,"
   but I have no heart for it.

My father's hearing, long since poor,
   has now gone bankrupt,
And even though I know
   this body cannot hear these words,
I finally say,
   "Goodbye."

Turning to my mother
   I offer words of comfort,
   though she does not require them;
      yet I persist.

It is one of death's demands—
   to engage in impossible tasks,
   to do what we must . . .
      lost in forgotten fields
      searching for a path away
      from where we began—
      a path with a new direction,
      toward a different destination.

And I am surprised to find my grief
   companioned by acceptance,
   as I stumble upon an oasis
   with a pool of sweet water
     where I rest a while.

Awakening, I am surprised to find
My hands clutching the holy grail,
   filled with a father's love.
One sip and I feel refreshed,
Ready for the rest of a journey
   that some say
   has no end and no beginning—
      to mend the hearts that never heal,
      to wipe the eyes of those we know
        who buried love
        and walk alone.

THE VISIT

It was sunny and warm that Friday
  when my wife and I were driving
  on winding roads, up and down hills,
  to see my mother,
Not knowing how many more times
We would follow this familiar route.

Firmly rooted in her chair
  but frail as a wilting plant,
  she greeted us with a bittersweet smile
  that seemed unsure if it would last.
    My sister made supper
      and mother ate some;
    Enlarged organs pressed against her stomach
    leaving little room for food.

Reminiscing through the evening,
  old times, better times,
My sister and I sang songs snatched
  from memories of mother
  as she played the piano
  and sang.

In a rare moment of silence,
  we heard a faint voice . . .
  mother singing one of the songs.
We had distorted the melody,
  confused the words;
  she set the record straight.

Time passed and mother grew tired.
My wife and I hugged her, said good night,
  and left her alone with my sister.
Walking up the street to my sister's house,
  the two of us passed
  through a narrative of shadows
  punctuated by streetlamps.

The next day we returned,
  but mother was missing.
    Her body was there,
      slumped in the chair,
      but her eyes were closed.

Inattentive to us and all else,
She seemed intense, as though
　focused on her weary lungs,
　　urging them on,
　　　the ebb and flow of breath
　　　signaling her success.

A necessary lapse, it seemed,
A need to be apart from us,
　for just a little while.

And soon a smile will announce
　her return
　　and her voice will greet us
　　with a laugh, perhaps,
　　　or a song.

As the day went by, the only sound
　was the faint whispering of her breath
　matched by the motion of her chest,
　　up and down, up and down.

She marched through the day
　with no seeming sense of purpose,
　　lacking direction
　like a wounded soldier, staggering,
　　eyes closed, alone, lost,
Not knowing where the road went
　or where it would end.

"*I don't know if there's a heaven,*"
　she once said to me,
"*But if there is I don't believe you see
　your family there when you die.
Wouldn't they remember the old quarrels?
Wouldn't we start fighting again,
　just like we did before?*"

I shrugged and shook my head.

"*I don't believe heaven is like that,*"
　she said.
　"*If there is a heaven.*"

But she was not talking now;
　she was barely breathing.

So we watched her,
   and during this watch
   minutes seemed to pause,
     while hours passed.

The watchers ate and drank and talked,
   and hoped that mother heard us,
   and knew that we were with her,
     but she was busy dying
     and did not seem not to care.

Before today, the deaths I've known
   have been long distance affairs,
     dialed up and delivered
     by a bodiless voice.

This was different, strange, unsettling.
Four of us imprisoned in flesh
   while one prepared her escape.
The watchers watched each other.
We stood, we walked, we sat,
   wondering what to do,
   listening to the sound of breathing.

Once mother exhaled and did not inhale—
   the silence stiffened our spines
   as we turned our heads.
My sister stood and walked toward her.
As if on cue, mother took a quick breath
   and let it out slowly and silently.

She was up to her old tricks again,
   trying to fool us.

More talking as we played cards, waiting.
I crossed the room and sat next to mother,
   taking her hand in mine,
   looking at her face.
The minutes passed . . .
   her eyes stayed closed;
   there was no response.

I focused on her face. It seemed stoic,
   yet revealed the rigor of her efforts.
The strain of breathing deepened her lines.
   A door in my heart opened long enough
     to permit pain at last to enter
     and make its home there.

The hour was late, and as I left I wondered
   what I would see when we returned.
Just past midnight, the phone rang.
   My sister said, *"She's gone."*
   And then,
      *"Do you want to see her,
      one more time?"*

Walking back through darkness
   to enter a room filled with light;
Still sitting in her chair, my mother
   seemed transformed beyond measure,
   startling me.

Neck stretched as her head
   rested against the back of the chair,
   mouth open, gaping, silent;
   no breath escaping now.

Her skin seemed to have shrunk,
   wrapped tight against her skull.

The stillness became a silence
   more eloquent than speech.
I was a witness to her leave-taking,
   a chorus of silent farewells.

Was it foolish of me to think it would not happen?
Was it foolish of me to think it would not?
Was it foolish of me to think it would?
Was it foolish of me to think it?
Was it foolish of me to think?

If heaven is . . .
   my mother should be in it,
And if family is not there,
   my father should be with her.

Having him beside her
would be enough,
   I think,
to give her the happiness
   she deserved.

SWING TIME

As she was dying,
She dreamed of swinging
   as a child;

Feet pushed upward,
Head tilted back to stare
   at infinite possibilities
   behind transparent clouds
   in a limitless sky.

The only grounding
   was the squeak
   and clank
   of the chains holding her,

Soon, that too
was gone.

                  Sally Sinclair

REFERENCES

Chief Aupumet, *100 Native American Quotes*. www.circleofexistence.com (select 100 Native American Quotes and then selected Chief Aupumet).

cummings, e. e. (1954). Since feeling is first. In *100 selected poems* (p. 35). New York: Grove Press, Inc.

Landor, Walter Savage. (1965). Death stands above me. In *Poems*. Carbondale, IL: Southern Illinois University Press.

Morley, Christopher. Christopher Morley Quotes. www.brainyquote.com/quotes/authors (Selecte "M" under the category of "authors," then "8," then selected Christopher Morley from the list of names).

Thomas, Dylan. (1957). Do not go gentle into that good night. In *The collected poems of Dylan Thomas*. New York: New Direction Book.

CHAPTER 6

Awareness: Promoting the Quality of Life

And come he slow or come he fast
It is but Death who comes at last.
Sir Walter Scott (1887, p. 54)

By telling stories about her family, my grandmother taught me that death could come at any time. She was born in the late 1800s and grew up on a Nebraska farm where her German and Danish neighbors "worked hard and drank hard." One of her uncles was six feet seven inches tall and weighed over 300 pounds. One evening he came back to the farm after a Saturday night of heavy drinking and passed out face down in a pigsty. He drowned in a puddle of water. "It took eight men to carry his casket," my grandmother said. "His grave was the largest one in the whole cemetery," and she smiled while she shook her head sadly at the waste of such a good, strong man.

Many of my grandmother's stories suggested that careless pleasure could have tragic consequences, and I remembered. Her stories taught me to be more thoughtful about what I was doing, and more cautious. I never assumed I was immortal as so many adolescents do. Once during high school while riding in a car, I was one of three teenagers packed into the front seat as my body pressed against the passenger door. It was dark and the road was not paved. The driver was going much too fast when he suddenly came upon a sharp, banked curve. He couldn't make the turn and the car slid off the road into a grassy ditch and rolled over a couple of times. Luckily no one was seriously hurt, but afterwards I would never get into a car if that driver happened to be behind the wheel.

> I adore life, but I don't fear death.
> I just prefer to die as late as possible.
> Georges Simenon

Like my grandmother, my father had an awareness of death, but in his case it was illustrated in certain comments or observations. Each time he had a birthday, for as long as I can remember, my father would always speculate on how much time he had left. For example, when he turned 40 he said his life was probably half over, but his tone did not suggest a dramatic despair. He was obviously prepared to enjoy the next 40 years as much as he had the first 40. When he was going through his sixties, his birthdays brought comments about having 20 more years, then 15, then 10. Although there was some sadness in his voice as the number declined, the primary message that everyone heard was that he was celebrating the amount of time that was left. Ever the optimist, my father's attitude about death seemed similar to the mathematical problem of the turtle having a big lead on the rabbit, but the rabbit reducing the gap by half each day. If the gap reduces by half, there's still a gap no matter how mathematically small. My father probably hoped that death would have no better luck catching up with him than the rabbit's mathematical chances of passing the turtle.

> Our common fate is age, sickness, death, oblivion. Our common hope, tenuous but persistent, is for some version of survival.
> Harold Bloom

Throughout my childhood and adolescence there were many opportunities to observe my father enjoying life. If the family was on vacation and went somewhere for lunch, he could walk into the most dilapidated greasy spoon of a place and find something to like. The quality of the food might leave a lot to be desired, but he would say, "This is really good coffee." I loved my father and have tried to emulate his love of life. Although my grandmother's stories tended to be cautionary tales about living longer by not making foolish choices, my father's example encouraged me to pay attention to my surroundings and to be aware of anything that could be enjoyed.

From these lessons I developed an awareness of death that prompted me to search for meaning and hope and joy in life. Yet I could also appreciate wry observations such as the response of famed economist John Maynard Keynes (1923) when asked about the long-term consequences of some economic policy: "In the long term we're all dead" (p. 50). Being aware of death does not mean accepting it and approaching the end of life willingly. I do not agree with the misanthropes who insist that life is to be endured until death brings it mercifully to an end. Furthermore, I cannot agree with pontificators who make speeches about "death with honor." Wilson Mizner (1979) provided the best response to such comments when he said, "Those who welcome death have only tried it from the ears up" (p. 138). No, I much prefer my father's example and try to enjoy life as he did.

> The more complete one's life is . . .
> the less one fears death . . .
> People are not afraid of death . . .
> but of the incompleteness of their lives.
> Lisl Marburg Goodman

People may believe in heaven and hell, or a paradise with virgins, or the peaceful oblivion of Nirvana, but no one knows what awaits us when we die. What each person does know, because you are reading this sentence, is that you are alive right now. To modify Descartes ever so slightly: you are reading and thinking; therefore you exist. Economic conditions, genetic limitations, and other factors can enhance or reduce an individual's options, but there are always choices to make. In some cases one's choice may be limited to an array of unacceptable options, as I discovered in the wake of my son's death. I wanted a world where my son was still alive—that was the only acceptable option, but that option was not available. At times an individual may be forced to select the least unacceptable option, but there will always be choices. Even refusing to choose is a choice. Other people are likely to judge us for the choices we make, and in that sense our choices determine not just how we see ourselves, but how other people see us. It is not likely that their perceptions will be the same as our own.

> Men do not care how nobly they live,
> but only how long, although it is within
> the reach of every man to live nobly,
> but within no man's power to live long.
> Lucius Seneca

Of the two poems selected for this chapter, "The Inheritance" was written for a friend who was only 47 years old when he died. Byron Meek was a colleague whose office was next to mine. We played racquetball together and shared many good times until he resigned and moved to Washington, DC. Years later, hearing that he had the HIV virus, I wanted to write to him but didn't know what to say. When he came back to see some old friends he met with me, and during our conversation I was surprised to find him at peace with life and with his death if it should come sooner than expected (it did). When Byron had to leave to meet some other friends, I shared my hope that he would continue to enjoy a long life, but he said he only wanted to stay healthy enough to enjoy whatever time he had left. This was the last time I would see him. Since Byron was not a religious man, his reconciliation with death was most likely a consequence of his deep appreciation for life. He cherished his experiences with his friends and family, and he simply wanted to enjoy the experiences he was yet to have as fully as possible.

> Cowards die many times before their deaths;
> The valiant never tasted death but once,
> Of all the wonders that I yet have heard,
> It seems to me most strange that men should fear;
> Seeing that death, a necessary end,
> Will come when it will come.
> William Shakespeare

Since Byron's awareness of death occurred in a secular context, the second poem describes an awareness of death from a religious perspective. For many people, religion plays a critical role in helping them respond to the death of friends or family members, although sometimes having a faith may not be enough. At a bereavement conference, I heard a Muslim father describe the loss of his son, admitting that one consequence of this death was that the father, at least for the moment, had lost his faith in God. The gospels suggest that the most enduring faith is that of a child, and that is the basis for the short poem that follows the poem about my friend's death.

Matthew (18: 3–4) explains why adults should believe as children do, and that was the inspiration for writing "A Child's Faith." The poem illustrates the simple yet powerful faith of a child—a faith that Jesus said was necessary to be saved. The poem began with the line "God is All in All"—a statement of faith with the same meaning whether it is read forward or backward. That line became the frame for constructing a sturdy box of a poem that would be impervious to the battering of doubts. The intent in writing the poem was to illustrate one possibility of what Jesus may have meant when talking about the faith of a child. To have a faith that can open the gates of Heaven, it must be a faith with simplicity and yet have the resilience to weather the storms of life.

Many examples from wisdom literature about the value of having an awareness of death would parallel Georges Simenon's emphasis on loving life instead of fearing death, and to focus on the need to live well if we want a long life. Harold Bloom sums up the dilemma of growing old as we cope with our physical deterioration while maintaining our intellectual hopes that something survives the death of the body. To this sentiment, Lisl Marburg Goodman adds that living a good life, or as she says a "complete" life, is the best way to overcome one's fear of death, and reinforcing her advice, Lucius Seneca suggests that living a complete life means to live nobly. He reminds us that we only have the power to make choices while we are alive, so an awareness of death should inspire each person to determine what constitutes a noble life and then to live it. Shakespeare goes further in a scene from Julius Caesar occurring shortly before his assassination. Caesar insists that fearing death fills our lives with fear; therefore, to live a good life we must live courageously in the shadow of death and not be consumed by the fear of it.

The essay concluding this chapter addresses the issue of what it means to create "A Culture of Life." The essay was written partially as a response to this concept as initially defined by Pope John Paul II, but also from hearing it parroted by prolife activists in the United States who seemed to redefine it. The concept of a culture that affirms life is appealing, but are Americans ready to embrace all the consequences that such a concept implies? Just prior to the execution of a murderer, a television reporter was interviewing a woman whose daughter had been one of the murderer's victims. The woman said that as a Christian she had forgiven the man for what he had done, but that she still wanted the state to execute him. Is there a place for the death penalty in a culture of life?

Many children in urban and rural areas are often hungry, attend inadequate schools, receive inadequate health care, and are given few options to escape poverty. Many die before reaching adulthood, and their deaths are recorded in our government's child mortality statistics. Many well-intentioned people object to abortion but they seem more passionate about the unborn than the suffering and dying children of the poor. Would a culture of life require a government that was committed to providing financial resources to these children and their families? Such questions need to be answered, and much would have to change before we could create a culture of life in the United States. The essay concluding this chapter argues that one change would be to cultivate an awareness of death to ensure a widespread recognition that every human life is to be valued.

The Inheritance

I was away all yesterday,
And did not hear until today
Of someone calling me to say
That Byron Meek had passed away.

"Passed away"—it sounds so odd,
As if, because the flesh is flawed,
It's "passed along"—en route to God?
(The message didn't say.)

But still I see his boyish face,
The six-foot frame, the shambling grace,
His gentle voice and firm embrace—
Too soon beneath the sod.

Yet from this source much more will grow—
His joy, his love will ebb and flow
Through cracks in Death's door—even so,
There is a vacant space

Which once he filled with raucous mirth!
How little time we have from birth,
And now this Meek inherits earth—
The poorer I, since he's below.

A life is done. What's left to say?
My friend was good, and grand, and gay.

A Child's Faith

God is All in All,
is for my best in
All His tests; man, All
in good time, blest is.
All in All is God.

A CULTURE OF LIFE

*We are such stuff
As dreams are made of, and our little life
Is rounded with sleep.*
                William Shakespeare

As we entered the 21st century, controversies surrounding the Terri Schiavo case and the euthanasia scene from the Academy Award winning film *Million Dollar Baby* prompted a number of Americans to express the need for our society to create a "culture of life," a phrase first used by the late Pope John Paul II. Although the Pope's use of this phrase would appear to encompass a much wider array of issues than those described by American exponents, the phrase itself is ambiguous enough to require some exploration.

First, we must assume that a culture of life does not currently exist in the United States since advocates are lobbying that the culture must change. This is not a new accusation, although it has not been widely disseminated. More than 20 years ago I attended a lengthy presentation by disability advocate Wolf Wolfensberger (1982) on the history of human services to an audience composed largely of human service professionals. At the conclusion of his address, Wolfensberger invited questions from the audience. Asked about his views on abortion, he bluntly stated that he found this practice abhorrent, in part because he believed that people with a disability were so devalued in our culture that if a pregnant woman and her partner were informed of a high probability that the fetus she was carrying would be born with a disability of any kind, the vast majority of couples would choose to have the fetus aborted. There is no greater injury to be done to people with a disability or any other human group than to deny them life itself.

Wolfensberger went on to make a more sweeping indictment of American culture by arguing that death is consistently chosen by Americans as a solution to problems, citing the examples of legalized abortion, capital punishment, selling weapons to the world and engaging in warfare. He argued that whether a problem was large or small, Americans frequently resorted to violence and death as their preferred response. In my home state of Wisconsin, people had been discussing the increasing number of feral (wild) cats in the state and the problems they were causing. When the issue was voted upon, the solution affirmed by the majority of those voting was to remove feral cats from the protected species list so hunters could legally kill them. The only thing that might have surprised Wolfensberger was the governor's declaration that he would veto the proposal.

Most Americans would probably reject the argument that the United States has a culture of death, but Wolfensberger's accusation startled me, and ever since I have paid closer attention to the kinds of solutions proposed in our culture to various problems. In one of her essays, "Life is Precious, or It's Not," Barbara Kingsolver (2002) reinforced Wolfensberger's concern: "(Our children) are growing up in a nation whose most important, influential men—from presidents to the coolest film characters—solve problems by killing people. Killing is quick and sure and altogether manly" (2002, p. 181). It would be a good thing if all Americans could be aware of such troubling comments and consider more carefully our responses, individually and collectively, to the challenges that confront us, to reflect on how we resolve our dilemmas. Each American ought to examine the moral and ethical framework that serves as the basis for making decisions, and all Americans ought to examine the consistency between what we say and what we do.

Many social critics have commented on American values and behaviors, and no doubt much more will be said and written. But to explore the meaning of a culture of life takes me to a different question: Is there a place for death in a *culture of life*? At first blush the question might seem absurd. A culture of life would presumably promote and preserve life in every way for as long as possible, whereas acknowledging death reminds us that life ends. Death is often perceived as the enemy of life. This perception stems from a fear of death that has haunted humanity throughout our history, yet there is another strand of that history, just as persistent, presenting an alternative view of death.

Literature from diverse cultures frequently laments the agonizing toil, pain, and suffering of human life in contrast to the peace of the grave. A passage from a book in the Apocrypha (Ecclesiasticus 11:28) illustrates this point of view: "Judge none blessed before his death." A major part of human suffering is to endure the loss of loved ones, but the commonality of this experience can become part of the consolation. After a friend of mine lost his adolescent son, he and his wife joined a grief group. The mother was moved by the stories of loss from other parents, parents whose children were murdered or died in a long, slow, agonizing process from a terminal illness. It put her loss and her suffering in perspective, helping her to live with that burden. She discovered the truth of a comment that has been attributed to Socrates and also to Solon: "If all misfortunes were laid in one common heap whence everyone must take an equal portion, most people would be contented to take their own and depart."

It is easy to become immersed in feelings of despair over the loss of a loved one, to see one's own suffering as especially painful and traumatic, but death and sorrow are part of being human. If people bring thought as well as feeling to such experiences, they may learn lessons far more valuable than what can be learned from a contented, pleasant, and untroubled life. Robert Browning Hamilton (1937) described such learning:

> I walked a mile with pleasure,
> She chattered all the way,
> But left me none the wiser
> For all she had to say
>
> I walked a mile with sorrow
> And ne'er a word said she;
> But oh, the things learned from her
> When sorrow walked with me. (p. 202)

My conversations with sorrow were recorded in my book about grieving over the death of my son. Shortly after *Sparrow* was published, I attended a grief conference in Canada held at King's College in London, Ontario. As an education professor, I had given many presentations at professional conferences, but presenting at this one created a lot of anxiety. The topic was not professional but personal. The audience members were not educators but hospice workers, hospital chaplains, funeral home directors, and other professionals who worked with grieving families and wanted to hear my perspective. I wasn't sure I could complete my presentation without weeping, and as it turned out I couldn't, but it didn't matter. After I had finished, one person thanked me for sharing my story, others began to share their own stories of loss, and their experiences established a connection based upon mutual empathy and compassion. I felt embraced by the 25 people in that room, and it was a welcome feeling for a man still struggling with sorrow.

This annual conference left King's College and is now held in Wisconsin. I still attend and occasionally give presentations. I continue to find the participants warm and accepting and compassionate. I have no doubt that there are people in attendance whose political, philosophical, and spiritual views are quite different from mine, but it doesn't matter because the people who come there have realized a simple truth that obliterates all the complex but ultimately petty differences between human beings—we all suffer and we are all mortal. On one level, such a realization may seem obvious, but existentialists have long claimed that the deepest appreciation for life can emerge only after someone achieves a genuine acceptance of his or her own death. Furthermore, many poets and philosophers have urged people to be less focused on and fearful of death and more concerned with living a thoughtful, purposeful life. As Victor Hugo (1887) suggested, "It is nothing to die; it is frightful not to live" (p. 276). Most people attending these grief conferences understand Hugo's comment because death and loss are so central to their work. Being so familiar with death, they appreciate the myriad experiences of life, good and bad.

People who work with bereaved families also know that grief is a life-long process and not a temporary state for a few months following a death. It is a feeling as abiding as love, if not more so, at least according to the poet Robert Nichols (1917):

> Was there love once? I have forgotten her.
> Was there grief once? Grief yet is mine. (p. 44)

Although Nichols is correct to say that grief perseveres, his comparison between grief and love is erroneous because he is confusing love with infatuation. Being attracted to a person may only last until aging changes the person's appearance (if that long), but loving someone transcends appearance to last a lifetime (if not beyond). Grief is equally durable, wearing down around the edges perhaps, softening over time, but kept alive by memories of the person who died. I continue to visit my son's grave and to keep him in my thoughts and in my heart. This grief will accompany me to my grave because my love for my son goes there also—the two are inextricably linked. Because they help survivors, people working with bereaved families know this. They offer these families the same empathy and compassion they offered me at that first grief conference, a gift that enriches both the recipient and the giver.

My most recent experience with death occurred a few years ago when my mother died. My son's death was sudden, unexpected, as shocking as being drenched in ice water while bitterly cold winds intensified the pain. Even though my wife, family, and friends were there to help, I felt isolated, physically weak, and emotionally numb. The journey through that suffering was slow and painful. My mother had a form of leukemia and her doctors gave her a range of time that she could expect to live. The onset of death became obvious when her organs became enlarged. She began to tire easily, was often short of breath, and she had increased difficulty eating as the expanding organs pressed against her stomach. My older sister became my mother's primary caregiver, but my wife and I drove down to visit as often as we could.

Near the end, her abdomen was pushed outward so extensively that my 84-year-old mother appeared to be 9 months pregnant. Concerned about the consequences of the obvious physical discomfort, one of the hospital staff asked my mother if she ever got depressed. My mother replied, "What would be the point?" When my sister told me about this conversation, we both understood why my mother would say this. She was already experiencing so much pain that she could do nothing about, why should she allow herself to become psychologically miserable as well? She would at least control the part of her life that she was able to control.

As my mother's body failed her and she knew her death was near, she did not fear it; she wished for it. My father-in-law had exhibited the same attitude when he prayed for death to come during those last few weeks before he died. They affirmed Stewart Alsop's (1973) contention that "A dying man needs to die as a sleepy man needs to sleep, and there comes a time when it is wrong, as well as useless, to resist" (p. 299). The last time I visited, my mother's wish was fulfilled. As day retreated into night my mother's breathing became more labored. Late in the evening my wife and I left after kissing my mother goodbye. Just before midnight my sister called to let me know our mother had died.

This was a very different death from my son's, and a different grief experience. I did not feel alone but part of a family; planning the funeral service became part of the healing and not part of the pain. This grief journey was an easier path to follow, filled with fewer questions, less pain, and more memories. My mother's experience satisfied conventional notions of how a life is to be lived with a beginning, middle, and end, not a life cut short abruptly at the beginning. There was a sense of closure here. My mother's life had run its course, and although she wanted to live longer, she did not wish to prolong the pain and the humiliation of not being able to care for herself in even the most basic ways. She was ready for death despite her own reservations about whether anything existed for her afterwards. In her last moments, I imagine her being prepared for this final experience of life, not knowing what to expect but ready for whatever would come.

I believe a culture of life cannot exist in the grip of an overpowering fear of death. That fear will destroy the positive attributes we should associate with a culture of life. It is probably impossible to eradicate the fear of death, but it can be diminished if we change the perception of death as a monstrous fate awaiting us all. As Socrates said, "No one knows whether death may not even turn out to be the greatest of blessings for a human being, and yet people fear it as if they knew for certain that it is the greatest of all evils" (Plato, 1956, p. 435).

If America is to evolve toward a culture of life, Americans must confront our fear of death and foster an acceptance of dying in the same way that we accept being born. Both are simply the processes by which we are brought into the world or taken out of it. What is more important is what happens in-between. Although my son's life was brief, it was not placid or uneventful. He experienced joy, frustration, romantic (unrequited) love, sorrow, intense pleasure, physical suffering, personal achievement, and psychological angst. He traveled with his family throughout the United States and traveled on his own to England and Germany. He left behind evidence of his personality and his aspirations in poetry, essays, and videos. I wish there had been more, but that was not to be. Life is given to all living things in different allotments as noted by Rabindranath Tagore (2007): "The butterfly counts not months but moments, and has time enough" (p. 438). The issue is not how much time we have, but how we use the time we have.

If Americans gained a new awareness of death and used it to promote a culture of life, what aspects of our diverse society would change? Perhaps less divisiveness between people, including conflicts that stem from prejudices. If so, that should lead to the end of segregation by race and class in our neighborhoods and schools. Affirming the value of every life means an affirmation of human diversity that would require the elimination of stereotypes so people could focus realistically on individuals, recognizing their actual abilities and flaws, giving praise for their achievements and helping them to strengthen their weaknesses. Recognizing the brevity of our existence could promote a culture of life transcending all historical differences that have been the basis for keeping us separate and suspicious and afraid.

Would a culture of life require everyone to believe in God? Belief cannot be required. Believing in any concept of God is a question of faith, and each faith takes a different perspective on issues such as the nature of the deity, the existence of an immortal soul, the function of an afterlife. If human differences are to be affirmed in a culture of life, then what would be required is respect for different faiths and for agnostics and atheists. What people of all faiths or none could agree upon is that each of us has been given an opportunity by being born. Life is an unearned gift, and to earn it we ought to consider what we can do to assist those who make this journey with us. As John Andrew

Holmes (1927) advised us: "It is well to remember that the entire universe, with one trifling exception, is composed of others" (p. 35).

Human beings are surrounded by life—plants and animals as well as human life. A culture of life should cherish life in its entirety. Native Americans expressed this in their cultures, but most Americans today have not yet learned the lesson. Human beings should be grateful for the opportunity to be alive and appreciate those we live among. Although we can never know for certain if God exists, we know that other people exist, vulnerable and uncertain, yet wanting to be hopeful. To cherish life means to understand the role that death plays amidst the flourishing life surrounding us. Plant, animal, or human life gets its place in the sun for whatever length of time it has, and then it is gone. The life we see around us is all the more precious for being temporary.

A culture of life would challenge us to perform random acts of kindness for people we meet wherever we are. Where there is suffering in the world, people stumble in its darkness. When individuals respond to suffering with compassion, it ignites a spark, and several sparks may combine to brighten a dark place. To create a culture of life in any society, people must acknowledge the inevitability of pain, suffering, and death in their journey together, and then extend to those around them empathy and compassion and even love. We must do this for each other and for ourselves. And it will never be enough. And yet it is.

REFERENCES

Alsop, Stewart. (1973). *Stay of execution: A sort of memoir* (p. 299). Philadelphia, PA: J. B. Lippincott.

Hamilton, Robert Browning. (1937). Along the road. Cited in Harry Emerson Fosdick, *Successful Christian living* (p. 202). New York: Harper Brothers.

Holmes, John Andrew. (1927). *Wisdom in small doses* (p. 35). Lincoln, NE: The University Publishing Company.

Hugo, Victor, Jean Valjean. (1887). *Les miserables* (Part 5, p. 276). In I. F. Hapgood (Trans.). Boston, MA: Thomas Y. Crowell & Company.

Keynes, John Maynard. (1923). *A tract on monetary reform* (p. 80). London: S. MacMillan & Company.

Kingsolver, Barbara. (2002). Life is precious, or it's not. In *Small wonder* (pp. 180-183). New York: HarperCollins.

Mizner, Wilson. (1979). *Peter's quotations: Ideas for our times* (p. 138). L. Peter (Ed.). New York: Bantam Books.

Nichols, Robert. (1917). Fulfillment. In *Ardours and endurances* (p. 44). New York: Frederick A. Stokes Company.

Plato. (1956). The apology. In E. H. Warmington & P. G. Rouse (Eds.), *Great dialogues of Plato* (pp. 423-446). New York: Mentor Books.

Scott, Sir Walter. (1887). Introduction to Canto II (Stanza XXX). In *Marmion: A tale of Flodden Field in six cantos* (p. 54). New York: Macmillan and Company.

Tagore, Rabindranath. (2007). Fireflies. In *The English writings of Rabindranath Tagore* (p. 438). New Delhi, India: Atlantic Publishing & Distributors.

Wolfensberger, Wolf. (1982). *The history of human services*, a presentation for Human Service Professionals at Madison, Wisconsin.

PART 4

Approaching the End of Life

For I have had too much
Of apple-picking: I am overtired
Of the great harvest I myself desired.
There were ten thousand thousand fruit to touch,
Cherish in hand, lift down, and not let fall.
For all
That struck the earth,
No matter if not bruised or spiked with stubble,
Went surely to the cider-apple heap
As of no worth.
One can see what will trouble
This sleep of mine, whatever sleep it is.
Were he not gone,
The woodchuck could say whether it's like his
Long sleep, as I describe its coming on,
Or just some human sleep.

Robert Frost
"After Apple Picking" (1967, p. 1067)

CHAPTER 7

Growing Old: Walking Through the Valley

> Let us cherish and love old age, for it is full of pleasure if you know how to use it. The best morsel is reserved for last.
> Seneca (1934, p. 67)

Although some people seem to view old age as a fearful walk through "the valley of the shadow of death," Seneca offers a more positive perception. Now that I have just turned 60, I would like to believe that Seneca's perspective is the more accurate one: that the walk could be pleasant and the shadows don't have to seem frightening. After all, most of my positive expectations for my life have been fulfilled. I hoped to marry and have children, and that happened. I hoped to earn a college degree and that happened three times. Although it was only a possibility as well as a hope, I assumed my children would marry and give me grandchildren. Above all, I was certain that my children would outlive me—I never questioned it, never even thought about it. My disappointments and frustrated hopes were minor until my son died in a car accident. His death almost 20 years ago now forced me to recognize that I could take nothing for granted, that some of my hopes would not be fulfilled.

> My old body:
> a drop of dew grown
> heavy at the leaf tip.
> Kiba

I recently retired, and like my father, I wonder how many years I have left. I have been grateful for the years past and will be as grateful for the years to come. The past years are not really gone, of course, because I can always revisit them in my memories. Now that I am retired, I have more time for such reflections. It is important to revisit the past, especially when you have lost people you loved. The only way I can be with my son, my parents, and my sister Gay is to recall our past times together. This gathering of ghosts fulfills my need to be with them, even though I am merely reliving old memories—previous conversations and experiences—rather than creating new ones.

Remembering past experiences with family and friends can provide a sense of affirmation of our lives. Not that every memory is pleasant, but they remind us that these relationships had deep roots that were watered with love. Even when battered by time, neglect, distance, and all the forces that can destroy relationships, memories give us a way to feel firmly connected. Remembering the times we spent with family or friends renews our love for them and confirms their influence on our lives.

> But there are moments which he calls his own,
> Then, never less alone than when alone,
> Those whom he loved so long and sees no more,
> Loved and still loves—not dead—but gone before,
> He gathers round him.
>
> Samuel Rogers

The more problematic aspect of remembering the past is the tendency to assess or even make judgments about our decisions. As people get older this seems to be a normal response to memory. In making these assessments we are also trying to understand the meaning of our lives; we want to answer the question: "What was my life all about?" Sometimes we may not like the answers we get, as British poet Sir John Betjeman (1954) illustrates in this reflective verse:

> There was sun enough for lazing upon beaches,
> There was fun enough for far into the night.
> But I'm dying now and done for,
> What on earth was all the fun for?
> For I'm old and ill and terrified and tight. (p. 43)

Many people appear to confuse the pursuit of pleasure with the pursuit of happiness, but Betjeman reveals an important distinction between them. It is difficult to sort out the meaning of one's life while you are living it, but it is reasonable, even necessary, to want to have some "fun" in life: to have vacations where you can lie on a beach or swim in the ocean, to celebrate with friends—especially on special occasions like holidays, birthdays, and anniversaries. It is necessary, but not sufficient. "I'm having a lot of fun" may be an adequate response during youth, but as we age it is not likely to prove a satisfying answer to the question: "What did I accomplish in my life?" And if the answer one gives to this question is not satisfying, then perhaps one's later years will be the time to do what finally must be done to provide a more satisfying answer.

> Don't complain about old age. How much good it has brought me that was unexpected and beautiful. I concluded from that, that the end of old age and life will be just as unexpectedly beautiful.
>
> Leo Tolstoy

Some people may not feel that their life was satisfying until they are older because aging can provide a better perspective for appreciating the past. Famed film actress Ingrid Bergman (2002) compared growing older with mountain climbing: "You climb from ledge to ledge. The higher you get, the more tired and breathless you become—but your views become more extensive" (p. 250). The views made possible by climbing that mountain may be breathtaking, but the beauty may be shrouded in ambiguity. The vista behind or before you may be beautiful, but what happens at the end when the climb is completed?

Lacking hard evidence to answer that question, many people reject the ambiguity by demanding certainty. Human beings in every culture have created religions to answer the unanswerable questions. These religions challenge us to have faith, to believe that the answers the religion offers are true, even though it is possible that they are not true. For some people that is not good enough. They find the ebb and flow of faith frightening, so they freeze it into a dogmatic block of certainties, condemning those who refuse to recognize their frozen image as "truth" and to worship at its altar.

A different kind of faith is presented in the song lyrics included in this chapter. They were written throughout the day on a Saturday in December, close to Christmas. Despite a heavy, wet snow coming down, I had to leave the house several times to run errands. When I returned from the first errand, melody entered my mind accompanied by the words for the first verse. More lyrics came after completing each errand, including the final one that occurred in the evening after the snow stopped and the sky was clearing. The first four verses describe observations from each of the four errands, and the last two verses are a general reflection on this quite ordinary winter day.

As the years pass and we come nearer to the end of life, we rely on our memories to assess and appreciate our lives. In "The Lost Mariner," from his book *The Man Who Mistook His Wife for a Hat and Other Clinical Tales* (1970, p. 36), Oliver Sacks describes a man with Korsakov's syndrome, also known as retrograde amnesia. In this case, the man's memory stopped in 1945, when he came back from World War II as a 19-year-old sailor in the Navy. His memory of his first 19 years of life was vivid, rich, and easily accessed, but he had no memory of any events that had happened since then. He could not even tell you what he might have done a few minutes earlier. Sacks described one occasion when he talked to the man, left for a few minutes, and after he returned, the man introduced himself to Dr. Sacks as if they had never met.

Some people might regard this man's condition as a blessing because having no memory of the recent past should mean that the man has obliterated anything painful that happened. Indeed, this 49-year-old man who believed he was still 19 appeared energetic and affable and seemingly happy; but he was not happy. During one interview, Sacks reported the following interaction:

> "How do you feel?"
> "How do I feel," he repeated, and scratched his head. "I cannot say I feel ill. But I cannot say I feel well. I cannot say anything at all."
> "Are you miserable?" I continued.
> "Can't say I am."
> "Do you enjoy life?"
> "I can't say I do . . . "
> I hesitated, fearing that I was going too far, that I might be stripping a man down to some hidden, unacknowledgeable, unbearable despair.
> "You don't enjoy life," I repeated . . . "How then do you feel about life?"
> "I can't say that I feel anything at all."
> "You feel alive though?"
> "Feel alive? Not really. I haven't felt alive for a very long time."

Whether our experiences have been good or bad, they define us and assure us that not only have we lived, but that perhaps our lives have mattered to someone. The short story included in this chapter was inspired, in part, by Dr. Sack's account of his patient with Korsakov's syndrome, but it was also based on my experiences talking with men who often made critical comments about certain physical signs that a woman was aging, especially their wives. They would point out the wrinkles, rounder hips, increased weight and gray hairs, while being apparently oblivious to their own physical changes. Although the narrative is meant to be tongue-in-cheek, it is also intended to celebrate the essence of genuine relationships, to remember what sustains relationships not only with spouses but with family and friends as we grow older. Such relationships are perhaps the best reason we will ever have to feel that life continues to be worth living.

> There is no old age.
> There is, as there
> always was, just you.
> Carol Matthau

Wisdom literature on aging often speaks of the rich perspective that can develop with age. For example, Kiba's Haiku evokes the fullness of a life approaching its final years. For Samuel Rogers, remembering loved ones is compared with a gathering of ghosts that revives your love for them (not gone, but gone before). In contrast to Rogers' bittersweet memories or Tennyson's description (below) of old age as a battlefield, Tolstoy speaks of the beauty and goodness he has encountered in old age, insisting that this is a harbinger of the beauty and goodness yet to come. Carol Matthau debunks the notion that old age represents a gain or a loss of our powers by arguing that individual personalities persist over the passing years. Finally, Tennyson's verse is among his best-known lines, and he challenges each of us as we approach our old age to remember who we are and what we stand for. He admits that old age may reduce our energies; yet he urges us to continue questioning and struggling and appreciating life to its end.

> Though much is taken, much abides; and though
> We are not now that strength which in old days
> Moved earth and heaven; that which we are, we are,
> ... Made weak by time and fate, but strong in will
> To strive, to seek, to find, and not to yield.
> Alfred, Lord Tennyson

Snow on the Evergreens: A Song

There's snow on the evergreens,
   the flakes floating down.
There's snow on the boulevard
   as I walk around.
There wasn't a warning, but still it's all right—
There's snow on the evergreens tonight.

The people all celebrate
   as smiles light each face,
And laughter is echoing
   their joy into space.
A sound just like music from mock snowball fights—
There's snow on the evergreens tonight

The streetlights are brightening
   a sky that was gray,
While winter is slipping on
   her white negligee.
A world sweetly sleeping, awaiting the light—
There's snow on the evergreens tonight.

And thoughts of eternity
   come drifting my way;
A single star telling me
   to treasure each day.
Though it's not forever, it's still quite a sight—
The snow on the evergreens tonight.

And just like the evergreens
   I'm burdened with cares;
The snows of these many years
   I'm privileged to bear.
As long as life lingers, enjoy its delights—
Like snow on the evergreens tonight.

THE MYSTERY

The love we have in our youth is superficial compared to the love that an old man has for his wife.
　　　　　　　　　　　　　　　　　Will Durant (1975, p. 50)

　　I am awake. Where am I today? Ah yes, it's a hotel room somewhere. I am traveling. And there she is, on the bed next to mine, still sleeping—the old woman.
　　Who is she? I don't recognize her. My wife should be in that bed, a beautiful woman who is young, like me, not this old woman with sagging breasts and graying hair and wrinkles. It is part of a mystery that I cannot seem to solve. Why do I keep waking up with this old woman next to me—sometimes in another bed, sometimes in bed with me! I don't understand. I want to see my lovely wife, but where is she?
　　Perhaps this woman is a companion paid to travel with me. But who paid her? I certainly have not given her money. In fact, I believe she has given me money on occasion. Am I being paid to travel with her? But why does she sometimes come into bed and sleep with me? Surely that's not part of my obligation! What is my obligation?
　　I need to go to the bathroom, so I get out of bed. In the bathroom I am confronted with the second part of the mystery. The mirror insists upon reflecting an image of an older man. It is not me! I am a young man with a full head of hair, vigorous and strong. I don't know this old man in the mirror. It reminds me of that Oscar Wilde novel I read years ago where the main character's appearance remains youthful but all of his sins and excesses are revealed in a portrait he keeps locked in a room in his house (and he has the only key). So perhaps this image in the bathroom mirror is revealing my sins, but what sins have I committed? I do not recall them.
　　This body of mine that should be slim appears to be rounder. Is that from the sin of eating and drinking? There are bags under my eyes. Is that from the sin of staying up too late and having too much fun? The wrinkles on my face must come from the sin of laughing too much. I see far less hair on my head and gray hair covering my chin, a few age spots there on my face. Do these signs condemn me for the sin of living too long? Such changes are not fair for these things are not sins! But I should not be upset because this whole thing is absurd. And I know that this is not what I really look like because I have proof—I have photographs!
　　If you look at these pictures of me you will see what I look like, a young man whose hair is at times long but sometimes short (I admit to a little vanity in trying different hair styles). Some of the pictures show

a clean-shaven youth, but once I enter manhood the pictures show me with a trim, dark brown beard (and no gray hairs). The photographs clearly document my smooth cheeks and my smiling, confident, youthful face. I know that this is what people see when they look at me. They see the young man in these photographs, not the image reflected in these pathetic mirrors. These mirrors are like the ones in a fun house, distorting reality for one's amusement. But I am not amused. I want to see myself as I really am, not this false image before me.

I return to bed, but there is the old woman again to reinforce the mystery. I lie down, trying desperately to remember, and some memories return, but they are vague. As I try to focus on them, these memories provide clues as to what will happen tomorrow, when morning comes. The old woman will get up and she will lean over my bed and kiss me, then she will go into the bathroom to shower. I seem to recall that sometimes she takes off her nightgown before she goes into the bathroom and I see her naked body. I think she does this on purpose. I think she may be attracted to me.

She has large breasts, I grant her that, large and round like ripe melons, but they sag because of their large size. When I have seen her naked I have also noticed her wide hips and fleshy thighs. They remind me of something, but I can't seem to remember . . . oh yes, the portraits I've seen in museums. You know, paintings of nude women lying on couches, their soft bellies revealing an appetite for food and pleasure. They are very sensuous, these paintings of nude women. I like them. Would I say that she is sensuous, the woman lying on that bed over there? Perhaps, I can't say. I think she has seemed a little sensuous when she lets me see her naked body before taking a shower. I only know that she is not sensuous at this moment. She is lying on her back, softly snoring, with the blanket completely covering her body. I really ought to investigate this possibility of her being sensuous the next time I see her naked. It will not solve the primary mystery, but it will be a pleasant diversion.

Wait, her snoring has stopped; her eyelids are fluttering. She is awake. I watch her stretch her arms. She rubs her eyes. She seems to be getting ready to get up. I am quite confident in my prediction about what will happen next. She will lean over my bed and kiss me—on the lips. She always pretends that it is a casual kiss, as if she is simply saying good morning, but I know that she is flirting with me, that she is attracted to my youthful good looks.

She sits up. Here it comes. I ignore her and pretend to look up at the ceiling as if I am lost in thought. She gets up and begins walking toward the bathroom. She did not kiss me! What does that mean?

Has my memory been faulty? What other mistakes have I made? Am I completely crazy? Is that the solution to the mystery?

Wait . . . she is turning around and comes back to my bed. She leans over it and smiles at me and then kisses me on the lips. When she walks away I can still feel her lips on mine, and when I close my eyes I still see her smile. What is it about her smile that haunts me? It seems so familiar. It is another mystery—a third mystery! As if I did not have enough mysteries to solve. I feel tired.

But wait . . . perhaps I may solve at least one of the mysteries. I am beginning to remember a woman who used to kiss me like that, and smile at me like that, a younger woman. It's all coming back to me now. I remember it clearly—of course, it was my wife! Every morning after she woke up she would lean over me and kiss me, looking at me just like that the old woman did. It was a look of love. I knew that look then. How could I have forgotten it? I think I would look back at her with the same look. Anyway, I certainly remember being in love with her, such a beautiful woman.

It is odd, but I think I love this old woman, too, in a different way from how I loved my young wife. But do I let her know that? Should I? Should I let her see a look of love in my eyes? I think I should. It's only fair. To be given such looks without returning them is like being a hoarder, a miser; it is like stuffing such sentiments under a mattress and getting no benefit from them. I need to remember this. I need to look at this old woman with a look of love, to let her know that I have some feelings for her. I know that this is the right thing to do.

But who is this old woman? What is she doing here? And, for that matter, why am I here? I wish I could answer these questions. As I think about them, it occurs to me that the old woman may hold the key to the answers I seek, but first I must solve the mystery of her identity. As I think about her, picturing her in my mind, I am beginning to feel certain that she is related to my wife in some way. I am not sure how just yet, but I think I am on the right track. I must not forget this. This is important. If I persist in my efforts to solve the mystery of the old woman, who knows, perhaps I will resolve all of the other mysteries as well. In fact, I am sure of it!

REFERENCES

Betjeman, Sir John. (1954). Sun and fun. In *A few late chrysanthemums*. London: John Murray Publishers.

Bergman, Ingrid. (2002). Quoted in Kathryn and Ross Petras, *Age doesn't matter unless you're a cheese*. New York: Workman

Durant, Will. (1975, November 6). Interview: For Durant, 90, history is in the past. *The New York Times,* p. 50.

Sacks, Oliver. (1970). The lost mariner. In *The man who mistook his wife for a hat and other clinical tales* (p. 36). New York: Summit Books.

Seneca. (1934). *Ad Lucilium Epistuala Morales.* R. M. Gummere (Trans.). Cambridge, MA: Harvard University Press.

CHAPTER 8

Anticipation: Preparing for Death

> *I inhabit a weak, frail, decayed tenement, battered by the winds and broken in upon by the storms, and from all I can learn, the landlord does not intend to repair.*
>
> John Quincy Adams
> (cited in Fadiman, 1985, p. 6)

Following his presidency, John Quincy Adams was forced out of retirement when voters in the Plymouth district elected him to the House of Representatives. In 1846 he suffered a stroke. Although he recovered and continued his public service, his health was failing. Daniel Webster visited Adams and recorded the above comment. In 1848 John Quincy Adams suffered another stroke. He collapsed on the floor of the House of Representatives and was rushed to the Speaker's Room. Two days later he was dead. From his statement to Daniel Webster, it would appear that John Quincy Adams would not have been surprised by this final stroke because he had already anticipated his death. Yet he was able to joke about God being unable to fix his deteriorating body and clearly accepted his coming death with grace and an unshakeable faith in his Creator.

How does one prepare for death? In previous writings I have quoted the following verse that was commonly used on tombstones in the 19th century:

> Stranger, pause as you pass by,
> As you are now, so once was I,
> As I am now, so you shall be,
> Prepare for death, and follow me.

These tombstones almost always have Christian images or symbols on them, implying that the deceased was inviting readers to prepare for death by developing or strengthening their faith in God, specifically in a Christian God.

Having such a faith is certainly one way to prepare for death, and individuals have chosen to follow different religious traditions that all provide a similar intellectual and spiritual preparation for death. Just to offer one example, here is what Mahatma Gandhi, a devout Hindu, had to say about death (1995, p. 14):

> It is as clear to me as daylight that life and death are but phases of the same thing, the reverse and obverse of the same coin. In fact, tribulation and death seem to me to present a phase far richer than happiness or life. What is life worth without trials and tribulations that are the salt of life? . . .
>
> For many years I have accorded intellectual assent to the proposition that death is only a big change in life and nothing more, and should be welcome whenever it arrives. I have deliberately made a supreme attempt to cast out from my heart all fear whatsoever, including the fear of death.

In addition, atheists and agnostics have written books and in recent years appeared on television to explain their attitudes about death. Rejecting the possibility of a divine being or an afterlife, many of them express a philosophical acceptance of death every bit as convincing as that of John Quincy Adams.

> Thus that which is the most awful of evils, death, is nothing to us, since when we exist there is no death, and when there is death we do not exist.
> Epicurus

All men and women must find a way to prepare for death because it is our final destination. Martin Luther King Jr. (1963) spoke of death as an example of a truly democratic process, since it was "the irreducible common denominator of all men," taking kings and beggars, old and young, innocent and guilty. The bigger question that human beings must answer is not how to die, but how to live. Death comes when it will come, and we are often unable to control the cause or conditions of its coming, but while we are alive, we do have some control over what we choose to do. If philosophers are correct in arguing that a good life is the best preparation for death, then each person must find answers to question: "What must I do to live a good life?"

This raises other questions: Who am I? What values are important to me? What have I said or done to reflect these values?

> I want death to find me
> planting my cabbages.
>   Michel de Montaigne

The loss of my son, a sister, and my parents has influenced my preparation for death. My grief process for them has involved emotional and analytical responses as part of an ongoing search for spiritual truths. This grief process could be described as a kind of "dance," but it is dancing without a partner. When others notice you dancing, you may become aware of their attention and feel embarrassed, anxious, angry, or depressed. You may even want the dance to end, but the music in your head keeps going, on and on. Over time you notice other people dancing without a partner, and inevitably someone comes up to you (or to them) and asks: "Why are you still dancing?" or "Aren't you done yet?" It can feel a bit foolish, dancing without a partner. Some dancers stop and walk off the floor, but others, a few, keep dancing. They try to be discreet; they move in and out of shadows so that they will only be seen occasionally. And a casual observer noticing them might wonder what they are doing, but someone else is likely to say, "Oh, he lost his son (or daughter or father or mother or best friend) a few years ago." Hopefully they will add, "Don't worry. He's all right. He just needs to keep dancing a little longer."

When we experience the death of loved ones, it is also common to ask difficult questions, and the answers we find acceptable will shape our thoughts about our own death. People may choose to believe in a God and a life after death. Some may commit to a particular faith while others develop a personal faith with an individual commitment that is not part of any organized religion. Some Christians, desperate for certainties in an uncertain world, have demanded a faith that guarantees salvation for believers, but in doing this they ignore the unequivocal statement in Hebrews (11:1): "Faith is the substance of things hoped for, the evidence of things not seen."

> Doubt is a pain too lonely
> to know that faith is
> his twin brother.
>   Kahlil Gibran

The final chapter of this book explores critical issues in preparing for death. Such issues cannot be presented as if they were questions in a multiple-choice test, requiring the selection of a single correct answer. Each individual must choose to engage in his or her own exploration, and in my case, because I was born and raised a Christian, this faith continues to attract me and influence me in ways that may not be felt by others. Much of my thinking about faith is not specifically Christian, but concerns generic questions: Is there a God? Are we immortal? If we are, what is the nature of the afterlife?

While some people believe there is no god, others believe in many gods, while many people believe in a particular God—a Jewish or Christian or Muslim God (and yet this is the same God identified by different names). Believing in a particular denominational God has never made sense to me. If God created the universe and all the life in it, why would this Creator designate a portion of humanity for special treatment and ignore or condemn the rest? I am not the first to ask the question. Thomas Jefferson and Benjamin Franklin believed in God, but rejected the idea that any specific religion represented the only way to find God. Even though they viewed Jesus as a great moral teacher and valued his principles, they rejected Christian claims about his divinity. For them and for many others, God was simply the Creator, and the evidence was the creation—the universe.

> Let children walk with Nature, let them see the beautiful blendings and communions of death and life, their joyous inseparable unity, as taught in woods and meadows, plains and mountains and streams of our blessed star, and they will learn that death is stingless indeed, and as beautiful as life.
>
> John Muir

As I continue searching for answers to my questions, I am haunted by the question Zophar asks Job (11:7): "Canst thou, by searching, find out God?" Perhaps for Zophar it is a rhetorical question, yet I continue with the humility of one who is deeply conscious of the many difficulties. If finding answers depends upon the sincerity of the searcher, then I can hope that my search may ultimately be successful.

Anyone's search, whether for God or faith or truth, is not simply a task for the intellect but involves the heart as well. The two do not always agree, but ultimately they must reach an agreement for the search to result in a philosophy or a faith that allows one to contemplate death without fear, either regarding death as the end of life or agreeing with the poet John Dryden (1979) who believed death meant "landing on some distant shore" (p. 136) There are many people who express such a belief, but others continue to be plagued by doubts and anxieties. Still unsatisfied, they muddle on, doing the best they can.

> Man is perishable. That may be;
> but let us perish resisting, and if it is
> nothingness that awaits us, let us so
> act that it shall be an unjust fate.
> Miguel de Unamuno

The poem for this chapter uses a format similar to one that the English poet George Herbert (1961) created for his poem "Easter Wings." Written in the 17th century, his poem is difficult for the modern reader, so there is a summary written in a format that illustrates the shape of the poem. "Easter Wings Resurrected" takes the wing shape and turns it upward or heavenward. The poem describes a Christian search for truth that ends by concluding that the answer to Zophar's question is "yes."

The selections from wisdom literature for this final chapter begin with Epicurus, who insists that there is no point in agonizing about dying since before our birth and after our death there is no consciousness to plague us with fears and anxieties. In somewhat the same vein, Montaigne's pragmatic advice is that the best way to prepare for death is to continue engaging in the activities necessary for life. For those searching for faith but plagued by doubt, Kahlil Gibran provides assurance that the one is related to the other, while John Muir argues that a close acquaintance with nature is ultimately the best way for all people, young or old, to understand that death is simply part of the life cycle. Like Muir, Miguel de Unamuno does not accept the finality of death, but in contrast to Muir he admits that this is possible. Even if death is the end, he still urges us to live in such a way as to have earned (and deserve to be rewarded with) immortality.

Although the essays that concluded previous chapters in this book were published elsewhere before being revised for this book, the essay for this final chapter was written especially for this book. "Wrestling with the Angel" does not provide answers, but it does describe a search for answers and some of the places this search has taken me. Hopefully the readers who are still conducting their own search may find something useful in it. As my grief journey winds its way onward, I suspect I have spent enough time describing it to others. I became a teacher because I love to learn, and my preference now is to spend more time learning by listening to the stories of others. In that spirit, it seems appropriate to conclude with words Benjamin Franklin requested for his gravestone, perhaps the final thoughts from his own search (Oswald, 1917, p. 237):

> The body of
> Benjamin Franklin, printer,
> (Like the cover of an old book,
> Its contents worn out,
> And stript of its lettering and gilding)
> Lies here, food for worms!
> Yet the work itself shall not be lost,
> For it will, as he believed, appear once more
> In a new and more beautiful edition,
> Corrected and amended
> By its Author!

In the 17th century, George Herbert wrote a poem entitled
"Easter Wings," an extraordinary visual poem
which begins by referring
to Adam's and Eve's "fall"
from grace but, acknowledging that with the
help of God, one's soul can still soar heavenward
(first set of wings).

In the poem's second stanza, the narrator goes on to confess his
individual unworthiness for heaven, as is true for
all human beings,
and he gratefully
acknowledges God's grace that allows him to
"imp my wing on thine" and in so doing enter heaven
(second set of wings).

The shape of the explanation (above) for "Easter Wings" duplicates the poem's shape. The poem (below) illustrates a Christian search for truth; the left side is to be read from top to bottom but the right side is to be read from bottom to top.

Easter Wings Resurrected

Oh Lord!	for Thee.
With anguished cries	within the mind
I search for signs, a word	the inward eye can seek
Before death dims my anxious eyes.	by outward vision—being blind;
Must I *believe* the prating pens of men	The love within my heart, not be deceived
Condemning humankind to lifeless end?	will it inherit earth . . . I must *believe*
When crucified, you died, they say,	for only if the soul is meek
And did not rise upon	my mortal weakness show
That Easter Day	these words I speak
At dawn . . .	But oh . . .

WRESTLING WITH THE ANGEL

> *To live is to wrestle with despair, yet never to allow despair to have the last word.*
> Cornel West (1997, p. xii)

Cornel West's comment concerns the pervasiveness of suffering in human life and argues that the experience of pain and suffering inevitably engages individuals in a struggle with despair. No one can choose to be immune from this aspect of life—the only choice we have is how to respond to suffering when we (or those we love) are confronted with it. People with financial resources may try to ease their suffering with material comforts and by the pursuit of pleasure, but that serves as more of a distraction than a solution. Others, rich or poor, have used some drug (or drugs) of choice—from alcohol to cocaine to heroin—to ease their suffering and diminish their despair, but drugs contribute to one's suffering and deepens despair. Although everyone suffers for different reasons, Cornel West believes that each of us can find a way to resist feelings of despair and not allow ourselves to be overcome by them.

The most significant suffering in my life came after my son had just turned 19 and was killed in a car accident. A few weeks after his death I wrote in my journal:

> Have you ever said, "I love you" when you knew the other person would not be able to say those words back to you? This is what happens when someone you love has died. It's a lonely feeling. You still say the words, knowing that nothing will follow but silence, and when you say them out loud you wait for the reciprocal response out of habit. You wait in silence for the answer that does not come, cannot come. You weep and you hope for a miracle, knowing it will not happen—demanding to know why not—feeling like you want to shout this demand to a deaf universe—shutting the shout inside, suddenly fearful of the answer to that demand.

Healing from the wounds of grief is a slow process. For years after Jason's death, there was still a persistent sensation of pain that could have me weeping at any moment. The power of that pain produced the following passage in my journal:

> Grief is a hole in one's heart—a black hole sucking in everything else that comes close, swallowing it whole, including your love for family and friends, your hopes for the future, and even your faith in God. If you're not careful, you may end up consumed by that

black hole, leaving nothing behind but an abyss that marks what once was a life, your life, a wholeness that was lost in a hole. When the abyss is all that's left, one's life will likely end by a cause, natural or unnatural. There is logic in this, for once a living force disappears into a void there is no being left to preserve, only a non-being that represents a horrific contradiction which cannot continue to exist.

For me, writing and rereading that passage clarified the importance of taking the process of grieving seriously and maintaining a consciousness of how that process was evolving. Since Jason's death I have watched one sister and both parents die; those deaths have been absorbed into the pain I feel over my son's death. The suffering from these deaths has not been due simply to the loss of loved ones but to the questions such losses raise, and with each death these questions emerge once again:

> What is the purpose of any human life that ends with death?
> Does the existence of an omnipotent God provide the meaning?
> Did this divine creator provide human beings with an immortal soul?
> If we have an immortal soul, where and how does it exist after our body dies?
> Does this afterlife include being reunited with our loved ones?

The struggle to answer these questions is like wrestling with an angel of death who refuses to provide answers. The essay's title alludes to the Biblical story of Jacob obeying God's command to return to the Promised Land even though his estranged brother Esau was living there. Jacob fears that Esau will kill him because Jacob deceived their dying father into giving him Esau's birthright. Upon entering the Promised Land, Jacob sends his two wives and children to make camp away from him on the other side of a stream to provide them better protection in case Esau comes to attack Jacob. The following passage describes Jacob's confrontation later that night with an angel:

> And Jacob was left alone; and a man wrestled with him until the breaking of the day. When the man saw that he did not prevail against Jacob, he touched the hollow of his thigh; and Jacob's thigh was put out of joint as he wrestled with him. Then he said, "Let me go, for the day is breaking." But Jacob said, I will not let you go unless you bless me." And he said to him, "What is your name?" And he said, "Jacob." Then he said, "Your name shall no more be called Jacob, but Israel, for you have striven with God and with men and have prevailed." . . . And there he blessed him. (Genesis 32: 24–29, RSV)

Although the angel gives Jacob a new name, there is no information about what sort of blessing Jacob sought or received in this encounter. The new name would suggest a change in his identity, and that resonates with me because when my son died, a part of me died with him. I may be a different man now, but this new identity is a consequence, not a consolation for my loss. Some people have tried to console me by saying that "God has a reason for everything." All right, then it is reasonable to ask for the reason for my son's death. Ever since Jason died I have been engaged in a wrestling match trying to uncover a reason for this tragedy, and the only blessing that I demand from my opponent is to give me an explanation. I accepted the death of my parents because they lived into their 80s and were able to enjoy life with their family and friends; even though my sister died when she was only 57, she had been a teacher for over 30 years and had touched the lives of thousands of young people. But my son was only 19. What possible purpose was served by his death? And if there was a purpose, why should it be kept secret?

This wrestling match has been going on for 19 years now, as many years as my son was alive. I have been given partial answers but none that are satisfying because they have not individually or collectively resulted in a final reconciliation with Jason's death. Although I often despair that these answers may be the only ones I will get, I am not giving up. This wrestling match will go on until I tumble into my grave, even if it largely consists of what wrestlers call "riding time," where few gains are made. I continue the contest partly from dissatisfaction with the answers, partly from a sense of habit, but also with a hope that the angel may yet offer a blessing that will bring peace of mind.

Of course, this situation is largely one of my own making. With a strong religious faith, I may have more easily accepted Jason's death, but I do not have such a faith. I have always admired people who seem to have a deep and abiding faith in God, but not those expressing dogmatic beliefs. The latter are too self-righteous and usually too judgmental of others to inspire admiration. Their self-serving certainties and the superiority implicit in their condemnations of those who do not share their beliefs would seem to contradict the meaning and purpose of faith as described in the gospels.

It is much easier to admire people who not only express their faith but live it; a faith so deeply internalized that they readily offer compassion to others. Such people typically refrain from making judgments; instead, they accept and embrace others, no matter what physical, intellectual or spiritual differences the others may have.

The God they believe in does not appear to be a distant and powerful entity to be worshipped out of fear but a constant and intimate companion in their everyday lives. I would like to walk with such a companion; perhaps this is the blessing that the angel could bestow on me. Perhaps this is why I persist in this struggle, although I don't expect to encounter an experience as dramatic as Paul's on the way to Damascus.

On the first day at a retreat a few years ago, all of the participants were asked to form a circle and sit on the floor. As a way of getting acquainted, each person was asked to share an important event in his or her life. After seven or eight people had described births or weddings or other important events, a young woman identified the day and time when she had "accepted Jesus Christ as my personal savior." My initial reaction to such statements is to be skeptical of people who make such a claim, especially when they use impersonal language as formulaic as this "born-again" mantra that I have heard recited many times by many people.

For the people at this retreat who were sitting in the circle, an immediate consequence of the young woman's statement was a sense of pressure on those speaking next to make a similar statement of faith. After all, hearing someone declare that finding Jesus was a significant event in her life made anything else seem trivial. Someone who had planned to tell the story about how much they wanted a puppy as a child and how happy they had been when they finally received one might now view such a story as rather mundane.

The next two people in the group hesitantly described their significant event. They sounded almost apologetic that their event might seem insignificant, but that it really was important to them at the time. Then it was an older woman's turn, and she said she would begin by first commenting on the young woman's statement. The older woman was not being critical, but she admitted to a sense of surprise at the young woman's ability to identify a precise moment for finding her faith. In the older woman's experience, as she explained, "God has just always been a part of my life."

The older woman went on to describe her significant event. I don't remember what it was, but I was convinced that she was sincere in saying that her faith stretched back in time as far as she could remember. What was perhaps most impressive was that her comment was clearly not intended to admonish the young woman nor to suggest any skepticism about her claim of having had such a dramatic experience. The older woman was simply saying that there were other ways to experience God's presence, that there were many alternate paths. In saying this, she created a more comfortable setting for those who had not yet spoken, and these people could now describe their significant event without feeling self-conscious that their experience might seem superficial.

Like this older woman at the retreat, the people demonstrating an admirable form of faith who have crossed my path have consistently engaged in behaviors reflecting a concern for others. This is an important point because it often seems that an individual has become a Christian only because of the promise of their soul's salvation. A frequent question I have asked of my Christian friends is whether they would still believe in Jesus without the promise of a heavenly reward? Would they still try to follow the challenging ethical principles that Jesus expressed in the Sermon on the Mount and throughout the gospels? Some have avoided the question while others—especially my friends who are ministers—insist that it's an unfair question. To ignore the resurrection of Jesus is to ignore the most significant single event in the life of Christ, one that is critical and central to Christian faith. Christians believe that by dying on the cross, Christ atoned for the sins of all humanity, and that the resurrection symbolizes the promise of a forgiveness of sins leading to eternal life. To ignore this promise of salvation is as unfair as asking Buddhists if they would follow the teachings of Buddha without the concept of Nirvana.

Fair enough, but I am still troubled by the world's religions. Why do Christians, Buddhists, Hindus, Muslims, and other believers insist that their faith is a peaceful faith, yet the followers of all faiths have engaged in violence against others? From what I have read, all of these faiths describe a special obligation to help those who suffer. Then why do faith-full people persist in the oppression of the most vulnerable human beings in their societies such as women, children, or the poor? It should not be too much to ask that Buddhists or Christians or other believers behave in ways that are consistent with the principles clearly advocated in the sacred texts of their faith.

Perhaps it was my rural childhood spent living in a small village that caused me to appreciate the ethics of the New Testament. My family did not have much money, and people even poorer than us were neighbors, so it was obvious that they weren't different from or inferior to me. The gospel's insistence on not judging other people but helping them always made sense to me. At one point in reading and thinking about the gospels, I was troubled by an apparent contradiction stemming from Christ's emphasis on being nonjudgmental but also forgiving. To forgive others implies a judgment of them; if one followed the mandate not to judge others, forgiveness would be unnecessary. Although the contradiction remains, an explanation that would eventually make sense of it was that the contradiction resolved a pragmatic problem. Jesus wanted people not to judge others while knowing that human beings were flawed and would still tend to be judgmental. So Jesus advocated forgiveness so that when his followers made such negative judgments, they could redeem themselves by forgiving others, and they could also ask for God's forgiveness for having been judgmental. To promote such behavior, Jesus promised that God would forgive the forgiving person.

Despite my ongoing attraction for the Jesus described in the gospels, I continue to be perplexed by a faith that emphasizes virtues such as love, mercy, and forgiveness, a faith that requires the faithful to share their resources and feed the hungry, house the homeless and cure the sick, and yet in the United States, where the vast majority of believers claim to be Christian, there has historically been a reluctance to do anything other than making token efforts to meet the needs of those who are hungry, homeless, or need health care. Perhaps it simply means that people belonging to the majority faith in a society are more attuned to the power of their majority status than to the obligations of their faith. Perhaps this is what Kierkegaard meant when he wrote about the difficulty of being a Christian in a nation that declares itself Christian.

Such thoughts and questions create the context as I grapple with the angel. Jason's death, and the death any child or young person, raises doubts about a God who permits the destruction of innocents, not only children but larger human tragedies, including the historic genocide against American Indians to the Nazi Holocaust to the death of a single child—including one who happened to be my son. The angel needs to explain how it is possible to believe that there is a God who cares about people and comforts them. On the other hand, I have received comfort in mysterious ways that some would argue was evidence of a God who offered consolation for my suffering.

In previous accounts of Jason's funeral, I described the incident where the door to the parking lot mysteriously flew open, banging against the outside wall, and how almost everyone in the family believed it was Jason's spirit leaving the ceremony. I have also described the dream that renewed my energy a week after Jason's death, and my cousin's dream with its message from Jason to read a certain page in the Bible (Psalm 84), which referred to the sparrow finding a home with God. Despite these experiences, my rational mind questions the proposition that there was divine intervention or that these events offer proof of the existence of God. They could simply suggest the existence of a human spirit that survives death, but perhaps only for a brief period of time.

Writing about these doubts makes me feel a bit like the person in the old joke who is trapped by floodwaters but prays to God to save him. When a boat comes along the man refuses to climb in because he says God will answer his prayers and save him. When a helicopter comes along he gives the same response. Finally he gets weaker and weaker and drowns. Once in heaven the man angrily chastises God for not answering his prayers and God says, "Didn't I send you a boat and a helicopter? What more did you want?" How much evidence do I need to believe in God? I don't know. Perhaps the only blessing that can be gained from wrestling with the angel is the blessing that the resurrected Jesus gave to doubting Thomas, blessing those who believe without "seeing," without proof.

Some people may rely on an intuitive sense of truth to make decisions about whether or not to believe someone or to take some action. My intuitive sense of truth suggests that there is a God and that each of us has an immortal soul, but the conflict of interest is so flagrant that my intellect is unwilling to accept this "truth" without challenge. Whenever this intuitive belief in God and my immortality asserts itself, a voice in my head insists: "You believe only because you want to believe, because it comforts you to believe." It is difficult to refute that allegation. The voice goes on to say that even though I may want to believe in God or human immortality, this does not make either proposition true or false. It is simply a belief. I have accepted the fact that the only faith that I will ever have is to choose to believe in the context of doubt, and such a vulnerable faith will require even more nurturing than a more robust faith if it is to survive in our tumultuous world.

If I force myself to be completely objective, I must acknowledge receiving some partial blessings as a result of a few outcomes stemming from Jason's death that have been positive for me or my family or others. Using donations from friends, family, and funds raised from the benefit performed by Garrison Keillor, enough money was generated to create a scholarship fund in honor of Jason's memory, and scholarships have been awarded to local high school graduates every year since Jason died. When Jan and I present these scholarships, we always tell the recipients and the audience of students and parents that the purpose of the scholarship is to support them in pursuing dreams that our son never got to pursue.

Another example: after *Sparrow* was published in 1994, it felt like a blessing when I received letters from several people who thanked me for sharing the story of my loss. A woman in Montana who had lost her son many years ago said in her letter that my book helped her deal with his loss. She also said her husband could never talk about their son's death before he died, and she wished he had lived long enough to read my book, because she thought it would have helped him talk to her about his grief. Her response was unique, but the following is representative of several letters I received:

> When I first started reading the book, I had a difficult time because I had not realized how powerful the book was. I felt as if I was experiencing your pain. Shortly after finishing this book, one of my co-workers died. Although we were not related, she enriched my life enormously and her death struck me very hard. Your book helped me to cope with the loss of this good friend. It made a difference in my life and I believe it can make a difference in other people's lives as well.

Writing about something as personal as the death of my child was a new experience. Prior to Jason's death I had written scholarly essays published in professional journals, but I could not write a book on grief using an impersonal, formal approach. In the process of writing *Sparrow,* my writing improved as I found my voice as a writer. I felt more confident writing my next two books; the third book, a textbook on human differences, has now become one of the most popular books in this field. Professors who use the book have said that a primary reason for the book's success is that students find the writing accessible and the complex ideas easy to understand. Many students have told their professors that they plan to keep this textbook in their personal library. I like to give Jason credit for this—that his last gift was to help me become a better writer.

Jason's death was the catalyst for all of this: establishing the scholarship fund, writing a book to help people grieve, and writing books to help people understand and appreciate human diversity. As satisfying as all of these achievements have been, I would trade them in a second to have my son back. Shortly after Jason died, I read a book written by a grieving father who was also trying to make sense of his son's death. He concluded that his son was taken from him because his Christian faith had diminished and God wanted him to renew his faith. That kind of thinking seemed surrealistic to me then, and it still does; nothing could fill the void that is Jason's absence. Nothing. Before beginning to write the first chapter for *Sparrow,* I wrote a note to myself about why this book could be a meaningful response to Jason's death:

> My son's life remains an unfinished tapestry with many threads hanging, a picture not yet discernible, too much is missing. What story would it have told had it been finished? A good story, I

hope, a satisfying story. Satisfying to me just for being finished, for that alone; especially if it were finished after mine was finished, after my loose ends were tied up and the final product hung on the wall for the children and grandchildren to see and say: "Whose story is that? Tell me that story." If I write Jason's story, that story becomes my legacy to my grandchildren, if they come to be, and to Jason's grandchildren who will never be more now than phantoms of my imagination, prisoners of a future that will never happen, frozen in time as surely as the dancers on the Grecian urn. Jason would have been a fine father and grandfather, so those phantoms represent to me an unknown beauty, an unspoken truth.

Despite the "blessings" just described, wrestling with the angel has taken a similar toll as it did on Jacob, who limped away from the encounter with an injured thigh. My pain has not been physical but psychological—a diminished sense of joy in life. It has required an increased effort to do what I used to do effortlessly—to teach, to be caught up in my students' lives, to be passionate about social justice issues. My favorite part of the book *Lives of the Twelve Caesars* by Roman historian and biographer Suetonius (1893) is the passage where he describes Emperor Titus at dinner, noting that he had done nothing to help anyone all day and concluding, "Friends, I have lost a day" (p. 471). Since Jason's death I seem to have lost many days by gazing more inward than outward, at times making me feel as ashamed as Titus for doing so little to help others. Yet looking inward has been necessary for my own healing. The challenge was (and continues to be) to refrain from becoming obsessed with my own needs. It is important to remember that helping others is not simply altruistic, but in the long run helps one's own healing process. Eleonora Duse (2007), a popular Italian actress from the late 19th century, expressed the need that human beings have for meaningful human connections: "When we grow old, there can only be one regret: not to have given enough of ourselves" (p. 187).

A final blessing should be mentioned, because it is not insignificant. Jason's death has helped me to prepare for my own. Jason would have wanted his family to remember him, but he would also have wanted us to get on with our lives and to enjoy life. We have done that, but the pain of his absence has been a constant companion. Like most people, I want to live for as long as possible and will do what is necessary to perpetuate my life, but my fear of death has diminished.

Some people think that the best way to die was the way my father did—at night in his sleep. It seems like a peaceful death, suggesting an easy surrender to what a French poet called "a great perhaps." At this point my preference would be to die as my mother did, surrounded by people who loved me, but being more conscious of them than she was. This permits a dying person to say goodbye to everyone, to tell them how much you love them, to feel the tug-of-war between life and death, and to fight that last futile battle. As the tide of the contest pulls me toward the impenetrable darkness, I would like to make the last decision that a human being can make—to recognize the momentum toward death, to acknowledge the end of life, and to acquiesce in that certain slide into oblivion with the love and support of those who are beside me, protecting me from the still grasping fingers of fear and doubt.

Honesty forces me to add that I cannot say, as my father did, that I am not afraid to die, but wrestling with the angel has taught me that there are fates worse than death. It is worse to die without having loved; it is worse to die without having lived; it is worse to die without having suffered since suffering can teach us about the limitations of being human. People can simply focus on their own suffering or they can use it to empathize with the suffering of others. Those consumed by their own suffering need to remember that they are not alone, and that there is evidence of hope if they are willing to look. Helen Keller experienced her share of suffering, yet almost a century ago she told us: "Although the world is full of suffering, it is full also of the overcoming of it" (2004, p. 130).

So I continue to live, loving life, yet recognizing that death is the inevitable outcome. I struggle with the evolution of a faith that continues to encounter doubt. As I approach the end of life, I hope I can retain my memories of the past while still creating memories in the present, and I hope my journey continues to surprise me with unpredictable events. Surrounded by others making the same journey, it is helpful to find those who are willing to tell their stories and to respond by telling them my own, because we learn from each other, and the stories simply make the journey more enjoyable. Like Chaucer's pilgrims, our stories illuminate our strengths and weaknesses, our joys and sorrows, our successes and failures. By telling these stories, if we are lucky, we will have gained enough love and compassion to light our way along a path that might exist in the darkness beyond the journey's end.

REFERENCES

Dryden, John. (1979). *Peter's quotations: Ideas for our times.* L. Peter (Ed.). New York: Bantam Books.

Durant, Will. (1975, November 6). Interview: For Durant, 90, history is in the past. *The New York Times,* p. 50.

Duse, Eleonora. (2007). Giving. In K. Weeds (Ed.), *Women know everything!* (p. 187). San Francisco, CA: Chronicle Books.

Fadiman, Clifton (Ed.). (1985). John Quincy Adams. In *The Little Brown Book of Anecdotes*. Boston, MA: Little, Brown and Company.

Ghandi, Mohandas K. (1995). *Mahatma: A golden treasury of wisdom* (p. 14). S. M. Ajgoaokar (Ed.). Mumbai, India: India Printing Works.

Herbert, George. (1961). Easter wings. In *The poems of George Herbert*. London: Oxford University Press.

Keller, Helen. (2004). Optimism. In R. Shattuck (Ed.), *The world I live in* (p. 130). New York: New York Review of Books.

King, Jr., Martin Luther. (1963, September 18). *Eulogy for the martyred children*. www.mlkonline.net/eulogy.html

Oswald, John Clyde. (1917). *Benjamin Franklin, printer* (p. 237). New York: Doubleday, Page and Company.

Suetonius, Titus. (1893). *The lives of the twelve Caesars*. A. H. Thomson (Trans.). London: George Bell and Sons.

West, Cornel. (1997). Preface. In K. S. Sealey (Ed.), *Restoring hope: Conversations on the future of black America*. Boston, MA: Beacon Press.

Afterword: Final Thoughts

According to the sources for these quotes, each speaker was lying on his or her deathbed or, in the case of Socrates, preparing for a dictated death. In some cases, the words here are said to be the last words the person spoke.

What is the answer? In that case, what is the question?
    Gertrude Stein

Now comes the mystery.
    Reverend Henry Ward Beecher

Now I am to take my last voyage, a frightful leap in the dark.
    Thomas Hobbes

God will pardon me. It is His job.
    Heinrich Heine

I am ready at any time. Do not keep me waiting.
    John Brown

I am going to seek a great perhaps. Draw the curtain, the farce is played out.
    Francois Rabelais

And now the time has come when we must depart: I to my death, you to go on living. But which of us is going to a better fate is unknown to all except God.
    Socrates

Index

Absence, living with an
  accepting the void, 63
  activities helping with, 66
  burdened, feeling, 63-64
  comparing grief, 65
  conferences, bereavement, 66, 67
  courage to go on, 65-66
  "For Those Who Stand and Wait," 67, 70-78
  "In Your Absence," 67-69
  not the person you were, realizing that you are, 17-18
  religion/God, 64, 76-78
  remembering as a way to heal, 67-69
  wisdom literature, 66
Adams, John Q., 127
"After Apple Picking" (Frost), 115
Afterlife, predictions of an, 19-20
Agnostics, 128
Alcohol, turning to, 54, 59
Alfieri, Conte V., 65
Anger, feelings of, 12-14
Anguish, emerging from the, 8-18
Apocrypha, 108
Atheism, 20, 128
Aupumut (Chief), 82
Awareness of death
  careless pleasures, being cautious about, 101
  "Child's Faith, A," 106
  "Culture of Life, A," 105, 107-113
  enjoying the time you have, 102-103

[Awareness of death]
  "Inheritance, The," 106
  loving life instead of fearing death, 105
  Meek, Bryon, 103-104
  misanthropes, 103
  religion/God, 104
  valuing life, 105
  See also Expecting death; Old, growing; Preparing for death

Bacon, Francis, 64, 66
Beecher, Henry W., 145
Behn, Aphra, 19
Bereavement. *See* Expecting death; Survivor, becoming a
Bergman, Ingrid, 119
Betjeman, John, 118
"Big Sisters" (Koppelman), 90-91
Bloom, Harold, 102, 105
Brown, John, 145
Buddhism, 18, 73-74

Caesar, Julius, 105
Capital punishment, 105, 107
Chaucer's pilgrims, 143
"Child's Faith, A" (Koppelman), 106
Cioran, Emile, 52
Compassionate Friends group, 59-60
Conferences, bereavement, 59-60, 66, 67, 109-110

"Culture of Life, A" (Koppelman), ix, 105, 107-113
cummings, e.e., 82

"Dance of Grief, The" (Koppelman), ix, 55, 57-61
Death penalty, 105, 107
Descartes, Rene, 103
Desires, frustrated, 5
Despair in check, keeping, 134
Dickinson, Emily, 48, 49, 65, 82
Dirge Without Music (Millay), 1
Donne, John, vii-ix
"Do Not Go Gentle Into That Good Night" (Thomas), 86
Dreams, 10-11, 74-77, 82-83
Dryden, John, 130
Durant, Will, 123
Duse, Eleonora, 142

"Easter Wings" (Herbert), 131, 133
"Easter Wings Resurrected" (Koppelman), 131. 133
e.e. cummings, 82
Eliot, T. S., 57
"Emerging from the Anguish: A Father's Experience with Loss and Grief" (Koppelman), ix, 8-18
Emerson, Ralph W., 21
Epicurus, 131
Euthanasia, 107
Expecting death
  "Big Sisters," 90-91
  dreams, 82-83
  "Holy Grail, The," 92-94
  indigenous peoples, 82
  Koppelman, Lois, 86-88, 110-111
  Koppelman, Roy, 84-87
  "Night Visitor," 82, 89
  poetry, 82, 88
  siblings, ones', 83-84, 87
  "Swing Time," 88, 99
  "Visit, The," 95-98
  what are we supposed to do with the information?, 81-82

[Expecting death]
  wisdom literature, 88
  See also Awareness of death; Old, growing; Preparing for death

Family relationships after a loss/death, 14-15, 18, 53, 63
Faulkner, William, 52, 55
Fear/death and a culture of life, 111-112
Feelings approach to the immortality of the soul, 20
FitzGerald, Edward, 63
"For Those Who Stand and Wait" (Koppelman), ix, 67, 70-78
France, Anatole, 23, 47
Franklin, Benjamin, 131-132
Frost, Robert, 82, 115
Funerals, 3, 11-12

Gibran, Kahlil, 129, 131
God. *See* Religion/God
Goodman, Lisl M., 103, 105
Grief journey. *See* Survivor, becoming a; *individual subject headings*
Grollman, Earl, 65

Hamilton, Robert B., 109
Heckman, Paul D., vii
Heine, Heinrich, 145
Herbert, George, 131
his mark (Koppelman), 24
Hobbes, Thomas, 145
Hocking, William E., 82, 88
Holmes, John A., 112-113
"Holy Grail, The" (Koppelman), 92-94
Hugo, Victor, 110
Human connections, meaningful, 142

Illness, Crisis & Loss, ix
Immortality of the soul, 20-23, 74-76, 88
Indigenous peoples, 21, 74-75, 82
"Inheritance, The" (Koppelman), 106

Intellectual approach to the immortality of the soul, 20
"In Your Absence" (Koppelman), 67-69
Ionesco, Eugene, 20, 22
"Jan and Tess, To" (Koppelman), 18
Jefferson, Thomas, 52, 53, 55
Jesus Christ, 104, 138-139
   See also Religion/God
Jewish mystical tradition, 21
John Paul II (Pope), 105, 107
Johnson, Ben, 5, 6
Journal writing, 3

Keats, John, 22-23, 48
Keillor, Garrison, 16, 17, 66
Keller, Helen, 143
Keynes, John M., 102
Kiba, 117
Kierkegaard, Søren, 20
King, Martin L., Jr., 128
King Lear (Shakespeare), 55
Kingsolver, Barbara, 108
Koppelman, Jan, 8-9, 11-12, 14-15, 18, 59
Koppelman, Jason. *See individual subject headings*
Koppelman, Lois, 84, 86-88, 110-111
Koppelman, Roy, 84-87
Koppelman, Tess, 14-15
Korsakov's syndrome, 120

Landor, Walter S., 21, 81
Life, a culture of, 105, 107-113
"Life and Death of King, John, The" (Shakespeare), 6
"Life is Precious, or It's Not" (Kingsolver), 108
Literature written by Jason Koppelman, publishing, 15-16
Lives of the Twelve Caesars (Suetonius), 142
Living, asking what is the point of, 19-20
Longfellow, Henry W., 54, 88
"Lost Day, The" (Koppelman), 5, 7
"Lost Mariner, The" (Sacks), 120
Love and grief, comparing, 110

Lucas, George, 16
Lucky Man (Koppelman), 23, 25-47

Making Sense of Death, ix
Mann, Thomas, 55
Masefield, John, 20, 22
Matthau, Carol, 121
Maugham, W. Somerset, 22, 66
Meditation 17 (Donne), viii-ix
Meek, Bryon, 103-104
Men Coping with Grief, ix
Mexican Americans, 74-75
Million Dollar Baby, 107
Milton, John, 4, 6
Misanthropes, 103
Mizner, Wilson, 103
Mohican tribe, 82
Montaigne, Michel de, 129, 131
Morley, Christopher, 84
Mortality, a consciousness of, x
   See also Awareness of death; Expecting death; Old, growing
Mother Night (Vonnegut), 73
Muir, John, 130, 131
Mystery, The (Koppelman), 123-125

Nabokov, Vladimir, 19
Native Americans, 74-75, 82
New person, becoming a, 17-18
Nichols, Robert, 110
"Night Visitor" (Koppelman), 82, 89

Old, growing
   accomplishments, analyzing your, 118-119
   appreciating the past, 119, 120
   Mystery, The, 123-125
   perspectives (rich) that can develop with age, 119, 121
   positive perception of, 117
   relationships, the essence of genuine, 121
   religion/God, 119
   revisiting the past, 117-118

[Old, growing]
   "Snow on the Evergreens: A Song, 122
   See also Awareness of death; Expecting death; Preparing for death

Pain/suffering and the preference of death, 22-23
Poetry, 82, 88
   See also individual poets/poems
Point of living, asking what is the, 19-20
Preparing for death
   Adams, John Q., 127
   doubts and anxieties, 130-131
   "Easter Wings Resurrected," 131, 133
   good life as the best preparation for death, a, 128
   grief process used in, 129
   religion/God, 128, 130, 135-143
   tombstones, 127-128
   "Wrestling with the Angel," 131, 134-143
   See also Awareness of death; Expecting death; Old, growing
Presence in your life, the deceased having a, 4

Quality of life, promoting the. *See* Awareness of death

Rabelais, Francois, 145
Reconciliation. *See* Absence, living with an
Religion/God
   absence, living with an, 64, 76-78
   anger with people speaking about, 13-14
   awareness of death, 104
   console using, people trying to, 64
   culture of life, a, 108, 112
   immortality of the soul, 21-22
   living, asking what is the point of, 19-20
   old, growing, 119
   preparing for death, 128, 130, 135-143
Remembering as a way to heal, 67-69
Rituals helping with healing, 59-60
Rogers, Samuel, 118
Sacks, Oliver, 120

Sandburg, Carl, 63, 66
Schiavo, Terri, 107
Scholarship fund in memory of Jason Koppelman, 15, 17, 66
Schopenhauer, Arthur, 81
Scott, Walter, 101
Seneca, Lucius, 103, 105, 117
Shakespeare, William, 3, 6, 47, 54, 55, 104, 105, 107
Simenon, Georges, 102, 105
Sinclair, Sally, 88, 99
Singer, Isaac B., 47
"Snow on the Evergreens: A Song" (Koppelman), 122
Social justice issues, 142
Socrates, 83, 88, 108-109, 145
Solon, 108-109
Soul, immortality of the, 20-23, 74-76, 88
Spielberg, Steven, 16
Spirit leaving the body after death, 12
   See also Soul, immortality of the
Spirituality/spiritual selves, 21, 74-75
Stein, Gertrude, 145
Suetonius, 142
Suffering/pain and the preference of death, 22-23
Suicide, survivors' thoughts of, 52
"Survival" (Koppelman), 54, 56
Survivor, becoming a
   alcohol, turning to, 54, 59
   "Dance of Grief, The," 55, 57-61
   denial of grief, 52
   exchange your death for the deceased, desiring to, 53
   family relationships, 53
   grief journey different for everyone, 51
   grief to take over, allowing, 53
   hopelessness that must be overcome, 55
   suicide, thoughts of, 52
   "Survival," 54, 56
   work/professional life after a loss/death, 53

Swift, Jonathan, 47
"Swing Time" (Sally), 88, 99
Tennyson, Alfred, 5, 121
The Fall of a Sparrow: Of Death and Dreams and Healing (Koppelman), vii, 17, 60, 140-142
The Man Who Mistook His Wife for a Hat and Other Clinical Tales (Sacks), 120
Thompson, Francis, 51
Tolstoy, Leo, x, 119
Tombstones, 70-71, 127-128, 132
Tragic Sense of Life, The (Unamuno), 21-22, 79
Transcendental experience, 21
Twain, Mark, 20, 88

Unamuno, Miguel de, 21-22, 79, 131
Unexpected death, an, 3-6

Violence/death and a culture of life, 107-108, 111-112
"Visit, The" (Koppelman), 95-98
Vonnegut, Kurt, 73

Webster, Daniel, 127
West, Cornel, 134
Whitman, Walt, 82
Wisdom literature, vii-ix, 6, 66, 88
   See also individual subject headings
Wolfensberger, Wolf, 107-108
Wordsworth, William, 4, 64, 66
Work/professional life after a loss/death, 9-11, 15, 53, 63
"Wrestling with the Angel" (Koppelman), 131, 134-143

Yeats, W. B., 8

SELECT TITLES FROM THE
Death, Value and Meaning Series
Series Editor, Dale A. Lund *(former Series Editor: John D. Morgan)*

STEP INTO OUR LIVES AT THE FUNERAL HOME
Jo Michaelson

LOSS, GRIEF, AND TRAUMA IN THE WORKPLACE
Neil Thompson

A COP DOC'S GUIDE TO PUBLIC SAFETY COMPLEX TRAUMA SYNDROME
Using Five Police Personality Styles
Daniel Rudofossi

FREEDOM TO CHOOSE
How to Make End-of-Life Decisions on Your Own Terms
George Burnell

PERSPECTIVES ON VIOLENCE AND VIOLENT DEATH
Edited by Robert G. Stevenson and Gerry R. Cox

WORKING WITH TRAUMATIZED POLICE OFFICER-PATIENTS
A Clinician's Guide to Complex PTSD Syndromes in Public Safety Professionals
Daniel Rudofossi

For details on these titles from the Death, Value and Meaning Series (as well as other titles dealing with death and bereavement), visit http://baywood.com.

SELECT TITLES FROM THE
Death, Value and Meaning Series
Series Editor, Dale A. Lund (former Series Editor: John D. Morgan)

DEATH AND BEREAVEMENT AROUND THE WORLD
Volume 1: Major Religious Traditions
Edited by John D. Morgan and Pittu Laungani

DEATH AND BEREAVEMENT AROUND THE WORLD
Volume 2: Death and Bereavement in the Americas
Edited by John D. Morgan and Pittu Laungani

DEATH AND BEREAVEMENT AROUND THE WORLD
Volume 3: Death and Bereavement in Europe
Edited by John D. Morgan and Pittu Laungani

DEATH AND BEREAVEMENT AROUND THE WORLD
Volume 4: Death and Bereavement in Asia, Australia and New Zealand
Edited by John D. Morgan and Pittu Laungani

DEATH AND BEREAVEMENT AROUND THE WORLD
Volume 5: Reflective Essays
Edited by John D. Morgan, Pittu Laungani, and Stephen Palmer

For details on these titles from the Death, Value and Meaning Series
(as well as other titles dealing with death and bereavement), visit http://baywood.com.